Adventures in Medical Writing

Publication Number 794

AMERICAN LECTURE SERIES®

A Monograph in

AMERICAN LECTURES IN
MEDICAL WRITING AND COMMUNICATION

Edited by

ROBERT H. MOSER, M.D.

Maui Medical Group
Wailuku, Maui, Hawaii
and
Department of Medicine
University of Hawaii
College of Medicine
Honolulu, Hawaii

Adventures in Medical Writing

Compiled and Edited by

ROBERT H. MOSER, M.D.

Maui Medical Group
Wailuku, Maui, Hawaii
and
Department of Medicine
University of Hawaii
College of Medicine
Honolulu, Hawaii

ERWIN DI CYAN, Ph.D.

Director, Di Cyan and Brown
Drug Consultants
New York, New York

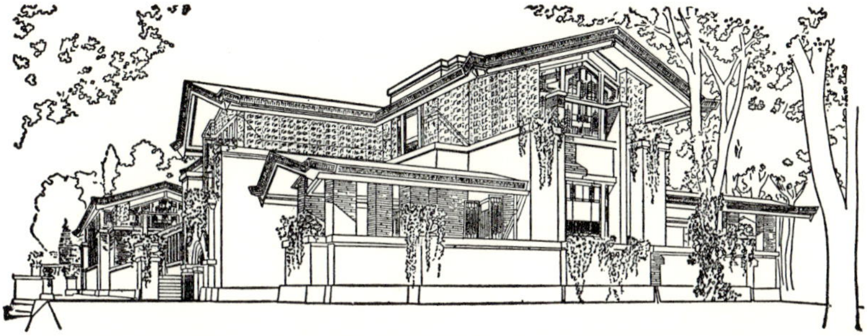

CHARLES C THOMAS • PUBLISHER
Springfield • Illinois • U.S.A.

Published and Distributed Throughout the World by

CHARLES C THOMAS • PUBLISHER

BANNERSTONE HOUSE

301-327 East Lawrence Avenue, Springfield, Illinois, U.S.A.

NATCHEZ PLANTATION HOUSE

735 North Atlantic Boulevard, Fort Lauderdale, Florida, U.S.A.

Library of Congress Catalog Card Number: 75–126486

Printed in the United States of America

K–8

Contributors

WALTER C. ALVAREZ, M.D., D.SC.
Emeritus Professor of Medicine
Mayo Graduate School of Medicine
University of Minnesota
Minneapolis, Minnesota

CHARLES D. ARING, M.D.
Department of Neurology
University of Cincinnati College of Medicine
and
Cincinnati General Hospital
Cincinnati, Ohio

WILLIAM B. BEAN, M.D.
Department of Internal Medicine
University of Iowa College of Medicine
Iowa City, Iowa

WILLIAM H. CROSBY, M.D.
Blood Research Laboratory
New England Medical Center Hospitals
and
Department of Medicine
Tufts University School of Medicine
Boston, Massachusetts

ERWIN DI CYAN, PH.D.
Director, Di Cyan and Brown, Drug Consultants
New York, New York

ROBERT H. MOSER, M.D.
Maui Medical Group
Wailuku, Maui, Hawaii
and
Department of Medicine
University of Hawaii College of Medicine
Honolulu, Hawaii

Foreword

The purpose of medical writing is to convey to the reader observations, experiences, or ideas derived from the medical sciences. These are practical purposes; they can be enhanced by good medical writing through clarity and specificity. Reading about medicine can be made a joyous experience through good writing.

In this book, we do not intend to teach medical or other writing. In fact, we doubt that it can be taught adequately, though it can be *learned.* Medical writing, similar to other writing, virtually writes itself. It is not a study but an experience which arises from study—after a writer has read widely, has become steeped in the power and beauty of the written word, and has paused to reflect. Thus, medical writing becomes a distillate of reflection.

It is not necessarily reading alone nor facts alone but their sentient transmutation that can make medical prose—or any other prose—a thing of beauty. Nor is it necessarily the product of writing courses. Courses can serve a useful purpose; they can help produce an acceptable, well-crafted product. But they do not strike a creative spark. While courses do not castrate your divine afflatus, they will not add to your fecundity. Facts and techniques *alone* are sterile.

To produce the substance of this book, we are joined by several contributors who, we believe, have something to say and can convey it elegantly and at times brilliantly. These contributors, Walter Alvarez, Charles Aring, William Bean, and William Crosby, are different facets of a gem. Hence, we are not disturbed at all that we may not represent a concensus. You cannot profitably argue as to which facet is brighter when you are warmed by the total reflection of a gem. Each of the contributors, including Dr. Moser and myself, takes up various facets of medical writing because we believe that the multiphasic aspects of medical writing cannot be encompassed by a single viewpoint.

Therefore, we commend for your enlightenment, entertainment, or enjoyment the variegated activity which is known by the omnibus name of medical writing, of which we offer a sampling in this book.

ERWIN DI CYAN

New York City

Preface

We are taught that there is a certain pride in creation. We know of otherwise timid artists who insinuate their names between the splotches of purple and marigold; sculptors are forever chipping their initials into toga folds. And authors usually sign their real names to poetry or prose of which they are proud (or at least insure that their agents give the pseudonym ample publicity).

It would seem, however, that physician-writers will launch a paper with blithe disregard for the fact that it would fail as a sixth-grade composition. And perhaps this is the hiatus in the links of logic—as one attempts to explore the reasons for the lack of literacy among so many physician-scientist-writers. Other essayists will pursue this point in depth. It is almost as though a *medical paper* is not regarded as a literary thing—as if proper syntax and grammar are affectations in a scientific paper. How this grotesque attitude ever got started would require deep investigation into the psyche of the medical scientist. (Perhaps guilt from recollections of a premature preoccupation with books —at an age when other kids were out playing kickball—has rebounded in some distorted gesture of defiance at proper English: "See, I'm not so bookish after all!") Or perhaps it is the reflection of an inferior general education.

My friends and fellow essayists will dissect this problem in far more elegant terms. Each has been carefully selected for his skill in medical (and other) writing and his outspoken attitude on this (and other) issues. And if *that* does not present a large, slow-moving target, one major thrust of this book will be dissipated.

We invite comment and criticism. Our hope is to enlighten, entertain, and provoke.

Each of the essayists will be familiar to students of the literature as a contributor whose medical scholarship is matched by his ability to record it in writing. Each has been "given his head" to pursue any tangent of his heart's desire in selection of subjects; variations in style and areas of interest make fascinating reading. Never have editors had to do so little.

The chapter order represents a feeble effort to present a smooth flow of subjects. Editors can have no favorites, but I think we have a "Beanean" classic aboard which may rival "Omphalosophy" as marvelous medical nonsense. Some overlap is inevitable, but it adds spice when one friendly toe steps upon another. We know there are many other superb writers in medicine, but there is virtue in brevity, and I think we have touched most of the bases.

So let's have at it!

ROBERT H. MOSER

Haiku

Contents

Adventures in Medical Writing

Chapter One

Nuts and Bolts and Assorted Gears

ROBERT H. MOSER

Before I pick up my spear to join the chorus—to deplore the state of affairs of American medical letters—let us listen for a moment to a voice from the other side of the aisle. Medical communication is not an art form to be admired per se for its elegance and color. We do not expect essays by Bacon or short stories by de Maupassant. We do not want cute, effusive prose—where one is obliged to take a machete to the semantic overgrowth in order to clear a path to the truth. We want the facts—uncluttered, unadorned. And I agree. But why not reasonable, inoffensive English?

Medical writing is a difficult business. Some of our more dreary trade journals remind me of poorly tended graveyards; one can turn to almost any page and stumble over bare, bleached bones—remnants of dismembered syntax, mutilated grammar, and neglected spelling—which are reminders of generations of witless, monotonous medical prose. It seems there is a feeling among physicians that good writing is an affectation—a manifestation of a frivolous nature, an unspoken sentiment that scientific data must be presented like chunks of parched jerky. It is my conviction that any reasonable analyst will assure the uncertain that there is nothing sissified about a clean-cut, well-scrubbed sentence; proper English is not a symbol of faltering manhood.

Writing a scientific article, however, is a project *not* to be undertaken casually. Each time you contemplate an addition to the sum of medical knowledge, a thousand years of predecessors are peering over your shoulder. Each time you append your name to a paper—any paper—your reputation and your pride ride in the balance. You are *laying it on the line* for all to see—for all time. The bad things we write seem to endure beyond all reasonable limits.

The integrity, depth, quality, and pertinence of your work will soon be judged. So, I exhort all who will listen: if you have something to say, proceed with caution; contemplate your project with care; execute it with circumspection; report your observations in good faith; derive your conclusions rationally; write it with clarity. And the scientific community will light a taper for you.

Mastery of the conventional literary disciplines (spelling, grammar, syntax) is essential, but perhaps of equal importance are attitude and philosophy. Writing a scientific paper should be approached like a military operation; detailed preparation and arduous conditioning are mandatory for success.

First comes the idea. Something has tweaked your curiosity. (I will not dally over false motives—such as the unspoken requirement to crank out a paper a month that seems to be a prerequisite for survival in some of our pressure-cooker publication factories.) But we assume your heart is pure and your motivation is genuine. A random series of events (experienced and/or read and/or overheard and/or divined) suggests to you that patients who are about to occlude a major coronary vessel undergo some peculiar perturbations of their pineal hormonal tides. Perhaps you tripped over this observation while checking circadian variations in pineal juice levels in two *normal controls* who then suffered coronary occlusions within weeks of the time you drew the samples. You would like to see if your suspicions have any truth. So, you ponder, ruminate, and kick it around with a few colleagues (and even with a few of the less hungry endocrine fellows). Is it sufficiently important to devote the required time, effort, and funds? Well, the *old man* thinks it just might turn out to be the hottest item since lipoprotein profiles and prepackaged martinis. And besides, Joe Hassenfeffer down the hall has agreed to set up a radioimmunodiffusion assay for your pineal juice fractions—for a small piece of the action.

Now you must determine if it has ever been done before. A preliminary scan of the coronary and pineal literature indicates that it has *not* been done or has not been done properly.

Next, you plan the strategy of attack—the design of the experiment. A great deal depends on the nature of your project. Were it a basic biochemical investigation of an *in vitro* phenomenon, or an epidemiological or actuarial analysis, or a drug investigation, etc.—all would have different rules. But yours is a clinical cardiological-endocrinological study—with its own particular set of problems.

Anyone who aspires to contribute meaningful new information to medicine must be tyrannic in establishing control criteria. (I will not delve into the delicate ethics of controls in the sense of elective deprivation of effective medication.) But at this point I would suggest you seek the help of some hard-nosed, steely-eyed, grey-headed type who has survived many years in the academic taffy pull. Perhaps he will be able to spot the statistical cul-de-sacs and deadfalls in your design.

I stress this because you must be prepared to exorcise any evil spirits of bias from your study. Enthusiasm is a pleasant enough virtue in newlyweds and linebackers, but it can be a devastating handicap in science, unless it is properly tethered. Perhaps the acid test of your integrity is to ask yourself, "Will I publish this report if the results are contrary to my expectations and the data looks like shredded wheat (and it makes me look like a bit of an ass)?" If your answer is *no,* I entreat you to desist. Your study will have intrinsic prejudice; it will take superhuman effort to expunge it later. Please do not add to the clutter which we all must struggle through in search of truth.

Well, by now you are ready to "review the literature." A proper survey will require great time and effort. So, you must set realistic limits. This is becoming less formidable a task in the computer age. If you have access to MEDLARS at the National Medical Library, send them a nice letter with the appropriate key words to facilitate the search. You want a ten-year survey of the English language literature on pineal hormones, hormonal effects atherosclerosis, etc. In a few weeks an incredible bibliography will be perched menacingly on your desk.

If you do not have access to MEDLARS, you will be obliged to employ more traditional methods. Your librarian can help you by plowing through the *Index Catalogue of the Surgeon General's Office, Quarterly Cumulative Index,* specific indices (i.e. *Excerpta Medica*), *Current List of Medical Literature,* tables of contents of medical journals, abstracts, annual reviews, and yearbooks. If you must tackle the formidable stacks yourself, it will consume much precious time.

But let us assume that friendly genies have plucked and harvested the pertinent literature for you, and now it stands in brooding piles: bound volumes, individual journals, books, abstracts, etc.—awaiting you in a quiet corner of the library. Each article you consult should be assigned its own 5 by 8 card with careful citation of author's name, article title, journal name, complete pagination, month, and year. You invite vendetta when you misspell a name, transpose or invent initials, or otherwise foul-up the vital statistics. One can often assess the character and habits of the investigator by checking the pertinence, accuracy, and timeliness of his bibliography—before reading the first word.

As each reference is scanned, notes should be jotted while recollection is fresh (use the reference cards if you wish). And please, if you elect to quote—be meticulous. Record every misplaced comma, split infinitive, and disembodied adverb. The wrath of a spurned spinster cannot compare with that of a misquoted author—whose magnificent prose has been dented or garbled or paraphrased.

Now the literature review is complete. And you are undiminished in your determination to stalk the cunning pineal humors. You probably started the bench and/or clinical work before the literature perusal was complete. In fact, as you became immersed in the project, new vistas came into view that required exploration of different avenues in the literature.

As you work, you are keeping detailed notes, creating simple charts and graphs whenever possible to keep the data clear. Periodically you are analyzing your information for accuracy and validity. If it passes your stiff muster each time, that often indicates the sound nature of your design, and you are commissioned to proceed. If not, you must fall back and regroup. It may require only simple modification before you continue. But if something has really gone haywire and the data are imperfect, or the controls have been fouled-up, or some menehunes have crept into the program, or statistical validation is *not* forthcoming—*stop!*

But, let us assume all is well—we have already established that your heart is pure—and the computer purrs in admiration for your splendid data. Now you sit down to write. Start by constructing an outline, with headings and subheadings. Most journals require a conventional format (*Introduction, Methods and Materials,* etc.) You may get an exception if you can convince the hard-headed editor that a modification will add to the drama or brevity of your opus. It also helps if he is your brother-in-law.

Now it is time, once again, to stop and review the situation. Line up the references, recheck the outline. Now say aloud after me: "What is the point I am trying to make? Did I make it? Is it really important? How did I prove it? Are my conclusions justified?" All okay? Fine. Now reach for your pen.

Begin with *Conclusions,* since this is where most of your readers will start. Here is the need for brevity and clarity. (It would seem you have proved that one of the more elusive pineal hormone fractions is at full rip tide for 7 to 10 days in the patient with angina pectoris who goes on to develop an infarct, while those with low levels do not infarct.) This astonishing conclusion, stated simply—without hedging—will insure you an audience. I would suggest that you check once again with *old steely-eyes* to see if he still agrees that your data justify your conclusions. You have done your homework; the design was sound, execution flawless, and you stand on solid ground. Now you can write the rest of the paper.

I prefer to tackle *Methods and Materials* next because it is so uniformly dull and so terribly important. This is where critic and defender will focus attention—to gather ammunition for assault or defense of your thesis. In this section the sagacious student can assess your experiment. And many a promising study has been aborted before it ever cleared the launching pad because of improper techniques, faulty procedure, sloppy workmanship, outdated or questionable methodology, and poor statistical mechanics. Do not let the small print deceive; it will be scrutinized. Take pains to reveal the nuts and bolts of your work—for all to see. This is a most essential component of your paper.

Next, I write the *Introduction.* This is the *lead* of your paper, and the laws of journalism are applicable. Describe *why* you elected to track down the mysterious second factor of the pineal hormone, *what* you are going to say about it, and *how* you did the study. (When and where have less relevance.) In the opening sentence you must have a "grabber" (a rather vulgar word borrowed from Madison Avenue, but it is appropriate in a sort of earthy, show-biz sense). You must intrigue the reader with a forthright statement of what your paper is all about. And if you doubt you can pull this off, perhaps you should reconsider the whole project.

Now you are ready for *Results:* a clear recitation of what you discovered. This is not the place for induction, deduction, inference, historical allusion, opinion, or philosophy. This is where your 2 and 2 add up to 4. No editorializing—just the facts. Do not repeat the dull stuff from *Methods.*

Discussion must be pertinent and logical. This is the *feature section* of your paper: the place for speculation. It is really the only part that permits much literary latitude. This is where you place your work in context—in historical and contemporary perspective. Inform the reader what hiatus in the total puzzle your work is filling or what virgin territory it is opening. How has your work modified or confirmed or denied previous concepts? It is here that you may feel obliged to *review the literature.*

Summary should be just that, not a tiresome repetition of what has been said earlier in *Introduction* and *Discussion.* It should be a pithy abstract of what preceded; it is no place for ambivalent weasel-words. Often, *Discussion* and *Summary* are lumped together, but I feel that each has a distinct function; I favor keeping them separate. It would be more logical to combine *Summary* and *Conclusions.*

Conclusions—we discussed this earlier; it is a precis of the *Summary*—in a few gemlike sentences.

A few words are appropriate about the laudable innovation in several leading journals whereby they print abstracts of the articles directly before the body of the text. Most of these are well done: a welcome device for the harried practitioner seeking "quick and dirty" information to assist in the decision to read or not to read a specific article.

Once I sit down to actually *write* a paper, I follow a compulsive little ritual. Being the world's least accomplished typist, I am obliged to do the first draft in relaxed longhand. So, I use pads of yellow paper (never white), legal length (never shorter), mounted on an oversized clipboard. My ancillary equipment consists of a cadre of fine-line, black-ink, ball-point pens; many ink erasers; a self-propelled contour chair (with an annoying, inextricable vibrator); three well-worn, carefully packed briars; and strategically scattered ashtrays, matches, pipe cleaners, spectacles, etc.

At my elbow I keep *Webster's New World Dictionary* (the unabridged stands mounted and ready in the library-sewing room), *Stedman's Medical Dictionary, Roget's Thesaurus, Perrin's Writer's Guide,* and Alan McGlashan's *The Strange and Beautiful Country* (to keep in mind how superb prose can be, when written by a poised, literate physician).

The first draft is agony. I "create" in the sequence described above. Reference texts, papers, charts, graphs, photographs—all begin in neat, soldierly files, but in short order, all is bedlam.

After the first draft I set the thing aside for a few days or even weeks. This is not done for any reasons of philosophic reflection or thoughtful appraisal but rather because I am bored with it. But I gird myself at a later date and reread it and modify it. In my more affluent days I dictated it on a belt and within a few days my secretary would present me with a delicious, triple-spaced, letter-perfect copy with two carbons.

Now, I am obliged to type it (wretchedly) myself. I give a second draft carbon to each of two aggressive (but bright) associates. We tear it to shreds (independently). This is a sadomasochistic little service that we do for each other; it keeps everyone very nervous but honest. Then I gather up the shards of manuscript and pride and write it for the third time, or I forget about it completely.

If this draft pleases, I lay it aside for forty-eight hours, and then I force myself to edit it again. I have done as many as seven drafts (some requested by those malignant pariahs of outrageous anonymity—The Referees).

There are some among us—heaven-blessed geniuses who more

likely have entered into some nefarious contract with the devil—who can publish after two drafts. They have my admiration and envy, but they are rare. Most of us are multiple drafters.

The technique of the writing craft represents a vast subject unto itself. Some writers are born, but for most it is a painfully acquired talent. To some it comes easily; others never learn to crystallize a decent paragraph. It is not a matter of intelligence, entirely, but I must confess, I have never met a truly educated man who was a total botch with the written word.

In my opinion, the best discipline for learning effective writing is *effective reading*. Read the classic authors; avoid the tasteless contemporary trash and explore the Great Ones. Expand your literary vistas beyond medicine; reach for those wonderful books gathering dust on the top shelves of your library—the ones you have been saving (for when?). Blow away the cobwebs and read-read-read.

Then begin to write-write-write, and then write it again. A literate (preferably nonmedical) friend can be a valuable sounding board. But do not wince and whine and defend when he lacerates your finest shots; it is a part of the game.

There are very few of us who can ever hope to achieve the literary magnificence of a Bill Bean, a Bill Crosby, a Charles Aring, an Erwin Di Cyan, a Walter Alvarez, a Jerome Lettvin, or an Alan McGlashan—but we all can do just a little better.

Finally, there is another facet of scientific paper writing that gets little public exposure yet provides abundant fodder for chart-rack gossip and well-counter intrigue: the ethics of publication. I suspect there are few things that can engender more purposeless passion among otherwise stodgy scientists than inept publication practices. And I have never understood what all the fuss was about. It seems to be largely a matter of proper manners—an ethic no more complex than good sportsmanship.

First, one must become familiar with the local ground rules. In some departments all papers (regardless of race, creed, color, or national origin) must be anointed with the *old man's* name as senior author. We all deplore this exploitation, but it is a real-life, frequently encountered aspect of the gamesmanship of medicine. If you singe easily, you can always pack up your columns and calculators and mortgages and wives and children and try to find someplace more civilized. There are many dandy rationalizations for this academic ploy (it *does* add to the status of your paper; it may hasten its acceptance by a *good* journal; after all, the *old man* did provide the atmosphere and stimulation that caused you to get the idea, etc.). But no matter how it is sliced or candied, it represents a form of minor piracy—but don't let it throw you. Swallow the bolus and finish your job; five or ten years from now it won't make any difference. Just be sure you do not play Lord of the Manor when your turn comes.

Early in the planning phase the potential author must consider *anyone* who had *anything* (of significance) to do with the project. Again, it varies with the nature of the paper. A case report would require that you speak to the referring physician, attending physician, house officers, radiologist, pathologist, etc.—anyone who made a contribution to the case. An epidemiological study would touch the epidemiologist, statistician, virologist, etc. Again, think who might be offended if you were to report this thing without talking it over with him.

Tell them of your intention to write the report. If they all say "fine," you may want to be a nice fellow and acknowledge their help formally in a postscript note. If you feel they should be co-authors, you must evaluate the degree and area of participation of each individual. The pathologist could review the postmortem findings and help select photomicrographs of key specimens; the biochemist may draft *Methods and Materials* (there is method in your generosity!), the senior clinician may help you with your literature review and editing.

However, if you tell them calmly of your intent to publish and they scream in outrage and accuse you of "stealing their paper" (which is always in its second draft and always has been accepted in advance by the *Journal of Exotic Minutiae,* whose editor happens to be your tormentor's brother-in-law), it is time for arbitration by a higher court. You refer it to your chiefs.

Now, this may turn out to be a friendly exercise by civilized men of mature judgment, resulting in a pleasant, productive, interdepartmental endeavor. It may hatch several versions of the paper: one for the pathologists, one for the endocrinologists, one for the cardiologists, and one for the little lamb that lives down the lane. Or, it can degenerate into a juvenile pout-and-shout contest replete with gallons of long-lasting, acrimonious nonsense. I have seen it go either way.

In the final analysis we are all practitioners of the Hippocratic arts, we are all more or less reared in the good old Judeo-Christian ethic, and we are all imbued from early childhood with the culture of good sportsmanship. And besides, what difference does it make if you have one author or ten authors on a paper? I will agree, if *you* are the principal worker, if it is *your* idea and *your* investigation, or it is *your* patient, you should stand on your flat feet and elbow your way to the front of the line. Your name should be first. But Smorgasborg, R. L. is really very little different than Smorgasborg, R. L. *et al.* when it is buried in someone's bibliography. Such generosity could save you much grief, and the people in Stockholm usually are smart enough to find out who really did the work.

One parting shot: if you had your masterpiece reviewed and blue-pencilled by a kindly chief (who does not eat his young), acknowledge him (and your secretary and technician and statistician).

Everyone likes a pat on the back—even a small pat in small print.

Chapter Two

Authors, Editors, and Referees

WILLIAM H. CROSBY

> External censorship of scientific papers is, of course, the function of the anonymous referees. Every professional scientist soon becomes aware of these mysterious deities, who must be appeased with all manner of absurd reformulations and sacrifices of beloved passages of text. In due course, he will be invited to take on this mask himself, and will roar like any ass in a lion's skin to frighten his junior colleagues. As you will learn at any laboratory coffee club, the editing and refereeing of journals is a fertile source of folklore, anecdotes, grumbling, and bad feeling.[1]

An old and malicious joke describes a passenger who wrote to the Pullman Company complaining of a bedbug found in his upper berth. He received from the company a most abject reply, to wit: all bedding in that car had been burned, the car fumigated, and the porter cast into the pit. But somehow the system had faltered. The passenger's original letter of complaint was returned along with the company's reply, and scratched across its bottom was the instruction: "Send the son of a bitch our bedbug letter."

Some years ago I told the story to a friend of mine. He had written to the editor of a journal after a quite good paper had been rejected. He pointed out that the basis for rejection, a statistical analysis of his data performed by a reviewer, was invalid because of a mistake in arithmetic. The editor's reply was emphatic—courteous but emphatic—in stating that his reviewers were selected from outstanding authorities of the world, each in his field, and because he himself was not an authority in this field, he was bound to accept the judgment of his reviewer.

Editors, like other busy officials, must employ form letters, and some entrust their secretaries with broad discretionary powers. I suspect that this particular letter belonged in the signed-but-not-read category and indicates misplaced discretion. In many editorial offices the decision whether or not to dust off a complaining author who is crowding the plate is retained by the editor himself.

These exchanges between authors and editors, between editors and their faculties of referees might be described as the backyard, or the backstreet, of medical writing. It is an area with room for improvement, and I suspect that any improvement in the quality of this writing would tend to improve the quality of medical publication.

The *Cumulative Index Medicus* currently lists about 150,000 titles per year from about 7,000 journals. These 150,000 represent the papers which are finally published, most of them after revision and many after the authors have shopped about, offering their wares according to a descending scale of editorial selectiveness. Editors of the "good" journals see many more "good" papers than they can publish. The manner in which they cope with the surfeit can affect the journal. Even the *style* of the flat-out rejection can make a difference. The routine rejection and even the routine acceptance is usually announced by a stereotyped but usually personalized note. The withering brusqueness of the printed rejection employed by the editor of the withering Yellow Journal just after World War II surely discouraged many authors from taking another chance. At this same time the Green Journal was beginning to be published and conducted its editorial affairs with promptness and courtesy. This, of course, was not the reason for the Green Journal's success. Indeed, the pampering of rejected authors may be considered time wasted, but it is one indication of the amount of effort and intellect that an editor spends at his job.

The editor's personality, aside from his index of indolence, also affects the nature of his journal. Some are adventuresome, others stodgy. Some editors permit their personal enthusiasms to dominate their journal's content; with others, their eclecticism prevails. Not for nothing was the *Journal of Clinical Investigation* referred to betimes as the *Journal of Milliosmoles* and the *Archives* was fondly called the *Archives of Almost Everything.* Some editors use an editorial board as window dressing, while others subordinate themselves to their referees to such extent that the editor's office functions as a ganglion rather than a brain.

Suppose two experts disagree when the editor sends them a paper for review. One replies "Great stuff. Publish as is. The attention of the authors should be directed to a common splice in lines 2 and 3 on page 32." This last demonstrates that while the referee does not know a comma splice from a copulative conjunction, he has read the paper carefully and critically. The second referee responds, "The experimental model is not valid. This has been reported in publications referred to by your authors (Nos. 2, 3, and 32). In those reports and in my own experience the method cannot distinguish between experimental subjects and controls." What is a poor editor to do? Accept? Reject? Read the references himself? Or take a vote? The ganglion-type editor may send such moot problems to a third, a fourth, even a fifth referee, seeking by a solid majority to express what? Judiciousness? Democratic ideals? Modesty? In the ganglionic editorial office where such polls are conducted, the quality of a referee's judgment may count for less than vehemence.

The good editor remains aware that a good referee, among his other virtues, possesses an ability to spot a lethal flaw which invalidates the most polished presentation just as he can discern true value camouflaged by a wretched presentation. In addition to his ability to find and exploit this virtue in his referees, the good editor should also sense any lack of courage or competence. He must remain alert against the referee who reviews serious work in a frivolous manner. Not necessarily the man who spikes his comments with wit or employs a pun to make a point this culprit does not put his mind to the job. A referee sometimes is confronted with a subject which lies outside his area of competence. Sooner than admit this or—God forbid—prepare himself by studying the subject, the frivolous referee fakes a review. "This looks pretty good to me," he writes, "but I would like to see them run another dozen dogs." (Never mind that dog experiments cost 100 dollars *per.*) Or he writes, "The authors have not measured the capillary diastolic pressure, nor the flicker-fusion rate, nor the postal DNA." And how is the poor editor to know that the recommendations are a fake or that the recommended work has already been done and published and cited by the authors? The referee who perpetrates this fraud doesn't know himself what work has been done.

> The trouble with some reviewers is that they read into an article what they think is there, particularly if they tend to disapprove of what they think is said. The trouble with others is that they do not wish to admit that they are passing upon a question they are not at all qualified to pass on. In any case, I think that a reviewer who rejects on erroneous grounds should be required to meet the objections of the writer without hiding behind the skirts of the editor. The present procedure protects the reviewer from tarnishing his advanced-degree rating but does nothing for science itself.[2]

Another sort of fake review objects to a paper on the basis of a subtly shifted objective. The authors have prepared a report on "Plethysmographic Studies on the Lower Leg of Normal Adult Human Males at Rest." Now, this critic really could find no fault with the report, but it would betray a trust were he to pass a paper without some measure of disparagement. So, he invents an experiment and then he finds that the authors haven't done this experiment; of course it is important, even critical: "The value of this study of the leg at rest will be significantly enhanced when the authors have taken into account the effects of exercise." The result: dust in the editor's eyes and salt in the author's wounds. The reason: to polish the referee's image of himself as the old Iron Duke. At this point the editor who is not helplessly indolent or hopelessly cowed by his own image of the old Iron Duke becomes an iconoclast.

This variety of editorial disorder has even occurred as an epidemic. There was once a scientist who had become so preeminent in his narrow field of competence that any editor who received a paper relating to that field would send it to this hero for review.

Now, it came to pass that nothing could satisfy him, nothing except agreement with his opinions, and deviation was grounds for rejection. And because the editors knew that he knew more than anyone, his word was their law. Some investigators said "to hell with this" and went to work in other fields. Meanwhile, the hero had no difficulty in publishing anything he wrote. By and by, some other scientists moved into his field with different tools, physics instead of chemistry perhaps, and they turned the old boy's flank, as it were. And it came to pass that all the work he had done was not so good after all, and no one sends him any papers any more. But while he was king of the beasts, he was able, with the editors' compliance, to put a stop to progress in his field for many years.

> You believe that you can contribute an idea worth considering by geologists, relating to the source of the forces producing continental drift. You submit a paper. The editor writes back that the reviewer has rejected it because you have no knowledge of basic engineering principles—"Everyone knows that the pressure in rock layers is the same in all directions." You reply that the reviewer does not qualify to pass on your paper and supply an exact argument based on elastoplasticity. Does the editor go back to the reviewer for a check? He does not, presumably because it would never do to question the reviewer's competence.[2]

The editor sits as the judge in a curious sort of court. The author is known, of course, and he must respond to questions put to him but without knowledge of his inquisitors, since tradition permits the editorial referee to remain anonymous. Equipped with this cloak, too many referees employ a dagger as well. Too many reviews are animated by jealousy and scorn and are degraded by insulting comment. The editor in his court may listen to an author's objections to this abuse, but he never finds the referee in contempt. Some editors who receive useful criticism couched in abusive language take the trouble to rephrase it before passing it along to the author. Others do not. On one occasion after I had refereed a paper, it was returned by the editor with this letter: "Our consultant, Dr. X, has just sent in his belated critique of the manuscript by Y, which you have reviewed. As you see, he takes a very dim view of the data. Does

Dr. X's slashing critique seem reasonable to you, and if so, would you care to change in any way your previous recommendation for revision?" I shall not report Dr. X's long statement, but it was of those which have been described as "little more than scurrilous personal diatribes, thinly veiled as scientific criticism." [3] I replied to the editor's note: "Thank you for sending me again the paper by Y. I don't have any additional suggestions to the author. Dr. X and I have said essentially the same thing in our criticisms. Only the style is different. I have no objection to your sending Dr. X my signed comment concerning his criticism." My signed statement read thus:

> Dr. X's first sentence intimates that the author of this paper needs assistance. His last paragraph indicates that the material is valuable and salvageable. However, the interposed intemperate analysis is of little value. It is an unpleasant example of abuse of the privilege of anonymity behind which we reviewers must perform. In order to salvage any part of Dr. X's critique, it must be rewritten to remove the insults and correct the spelling. For this reason his performance is as incompetent as that of the authors whom he assails. Instead of sneering at another reviewer's kindness, he might better have accepted the role of friendly counsellor and offered this author the benefit of his insights and wisdom in a form which he could accept to improve the work and thereby benefit us all.

I learned later that the editor sent my signed statement not to Dr. X the referee but to Dr. Y the author, together with X's diatribe. Y repaired his paper, and it was published, but what of the plight of poor Dr. X? If his editor won't tell him about Listerine, who will ever do it?

From time to time at the meetings of editorial boards, I have asked that we abandon the anonymity of referees. The response to this suggestion is always the same. Imagine me as the hunchbacked Quasimodo swinging aloft amidst the clashing bells in the tower of Notre Dame and you will have some inkling of the vigor of the board's reaction to this modest proposal. The substance is their reaction was "Terrible! That would deprive us of our freedom of expression." What they really mean is their freedom to write sloppy, off-the-top-of-the-head, emotional, undocumented, unchallengeable reviews. When entrenched privilege feels threatened, there is always a right or a freedom which must be defended. Abolition of slavery was attacked as an infringement of property rights.

Humanity adjusts to evil. For generations civilizations have blandly permitted, even insisted upon, such horrors as infanticide, ritual sacrifice, cannibalism, war, and no salary for interns. In the scale of wickedness the anonymity of referees does not rate high, perhaps a little above the disenfranchisement of women, but it is an evil which the scientific community has tolerated too long with unwholesome permissiveness. Among countless victims of the system only an occasional author has had to receive an exemplary flogging for rebellion. But the winds of change are blowing. A system based upon human misery cannot survive in our free society. This relic of nineteenth century professorial gamesmanship, this too shall pass away.

References

1. Ziman, J. M.: Information, communication, knowledge. *Nature 224:*318–324, 1969.
2. Richardson, E. A.: Authors, editors and referees. *Science 124:* 443–444, 1965.
3. Page, I. H.: Needless pains caused by heedless editors. *Science 123:*1241, 1965.

Chapter Three

Thoughts and Things on Medical Writings

ERWIN DI CYAN

Writing is an act of faith, not a trick of grammar.
——E. B. WHITE

ON THE TONE OF THE TEXT

WE SEEM to be overoccupied with the nuts and bolts of medical writing, while the big problems lie elsewhere than in its hardware. The problem lies in the emotional wasteland—in the tone; we have a fertile language which is being desiccated by arid writers. It is as if the scientist or physician-writer must first emasculate all emotions of his speech, or of his paper, before it will confer status on him.

Most people have been brainwashed into believing that it is disgraceful to feel. Practice makes it so. The medical writer, in common with other people in our times, is beset with an alienation of many affects and often stumbles when he attempts to express himself naturally. Natural speech is colorful—or should be so—because of its emotional content.

As a matter of professional need, we must read and study much of the current medical or other scientific literature. An activity which should be pleasuresome as well as useful, I confess, becomes, at times, quite boring.

Why should this happen? I believe that the principal reason

lies in the monotony, the utter lack of humor, the sameness of most items. The subjects may differ, but the words are rigidly encased in the same drab uniform.

Everyone recognizes, I assume, that monotony produces boredom. This is a fact of life, whether it be the same dish that is put before you daily, or the same inane activity that you perform without variation, or the same mawkish stuff that you read. For example, to avoid monotony, a clever hostess often puts a piquant note into her dinner parties—whether it is a different dish, or a different group of guests, or even a variety of colors or a change in the shape of the *hors d'oeuvres*. You forget the commonly flat taste of most *hors d'oeuvres* when there is a variety in shape or color—which should change frequently in order to preserve the stimulus of variety.

The author of the scientific paper puts the same ordure into his verdure. The words are rearranged from paper to paper, the subjects change, and the reported results may be different, but the same chill of unimaginative and impersonal prose enhulls you because the stuff is so prosaic and impersonal.

It appears to me that if the alienated author were to share with the reader what process, observation, etc., sparked his curiosity to undertake the work that he so nobly if boringly reports, he may give the reader a broader insight; it may prove to be of heuristic usefulness. We talk about the need for communication—yet, how well do we communicate?

Does the average researcher never spontaneously stop to wonder at the enormity of the system or the majesty of the functions on which he reports his little findings? If he does not, he is indeed average; if he does, why is he ashamed to share his spontaneous reaction with his readers?

Have we also lost our sense of humor? My question is really rhetorical because I am reasonably convinced that humor is in eclipse together with a natural manner of expressing ourselves as well as any expression of emotion or of insight. Seven-letter words—like emotion or insight—seem to be banished as four letter words once were! We seem to be ashamed of writing in any way except in a monotonous, wooden recitation with no modulation. Apparently, we believe that the latter belongs to the era of antimacassars or perhaps in the British medical and scientific literature?

Surely, not everything in a given paper is of equal importance. Does it not appear reasonable, therefore, to modulate our prose and convey to the reader in a live way—somewhat like the British medical and scientific journals do? Would we ever think of delivering a talk in the colorless and monotonous way that many of us write? I had forgotten, the talks do sound the same way!

That is the reason most of us avoid them!

ON DISEASES OF PROSE

Prose has its diseases. They are probably contagious, for how else can we account for the epidemic spread of writing dysfunctions—especially dysfunctions of scientific writing?

A minor and rather unimportant disease is *ptosis*—exemplified by such symptoms as a dropped comma. An even less important dysfunction presents occasional split infinitives as the principal symptoms. But because of its wider ramifications there is a more important disease called *thesauropifflosis*—a contraction of *thesaurosis* and *piffle*—which has as its principal symptom a storing up and an overconcern with trivia. With the increasing importance of the computer, that condition is increasing.

A prose disease of equally great importance is *double-entendry*—derived from *double* and *entendre*. In it, a statement presumably expresses what the writer wished to convey but allows—even presses—the reader to infer an additional or collateral meaning not intended by the writer. Here is an example: "As a result of the clinical experience, it was postulated that these pregnancies resulted from an imbalance between instinctual drives and motivation, on the one hand, and self-control on the other." Inferentially, some readers may inquire what happened to the old wives' fable about pregnancy resulting from coitus?

A similar statement, seriously intended, is found in David Seabury's *The Art of Selfishness* (1937): "I know a boy who ran with wild companions until he realized that the diseases he might get could infect his home and might do injury to his mother and sisters." Some readers may inquire if this was an incestuous house.

Since we are speaking of meanings—instead of periods and commas—we should explore another disease of prose, namely *cryptographia.* Prose afflicted with this condition hides a specific meaning from the reader either by vagueness, generality, or by some vapid device which precludes a clear view of what happened. For example, in a report of an unusual case, the writer tells us that he discovered the reported findings in a patient after the patient ". . . was admitted for an unrelated disorder." If the case is so unusual as to merit publication in a fine journal, perhaps the *unrelated disorder* may not be so unrelated—let the reader decide that. Imperious shedding of *unrelated disorders* does violence to future searches in the literature. For example, urethritis and conjunctivitis are quite unrelated to arthritis. Yet a triad Reiter's disease was discovered by correlating these seemingly unrelated three symptoms. Another example resides in the association of thyroid disease with the subsequent development of a lymphatic disorder. Perhaps this association of entities was found only because early writers on lymphatic diseases did not summarily conclude that an admission resulting from thyroid disease was unrelated to a lymphatic disease, and they left the question open.

A similar condition is *hermaphrographia.* Prose afflicted with it does not specify which is which, i.e., whether an event is up or down or to what side it leans. An example is a digest report that the prothrombin level is *altered* or *affected* in persons taking phenobarbital. But how? Is the prothrombin level depressed or exaggerated or can it be altered in either direction? The same disease of prose is responsible for such expressions in a summary as ". . . has an effect on oxidative phosphorylation" (does it uncouple it, hinder it, stimulate it?), or "changes were observed" (what changes?), or ". . . the fatigue appears to be linked with changes in the enzyme levels" (fatigue of what? muscle fatigue or just subjective feeling of fatigue?). In the same vein, the reader learns in the digest of another article that ". . . there is no established rationale for the use of *x* in the relief of pruritus associated with other disease processes," but he never finds out if *x* has been tried and found wanting or if it has just not yet been tried in the ". . . pruritus associated with other disease processes."

Diseases of prose often respond to demonstration: the prose improves or its dysfunctions may be cured when they are pointed out to the writer. While a new specialist—the *graphonosologist,* one who specializes in classifying diseases of prose—is arising in response to the increased incidence of diseases of prose, his services are usually not necessary for therapy because the remedies for diseases of prose are available over-the-counter. That is usually the book counter; it sells many books freed from diseases of prose. They may be taken as necessary—their only side effect is the inroads they make on available time and cash.

ON STUFFY NOTATIONS

Scholars and pedants copiously use abbreviated, bibliographic notations in manuscript or text. I wouldn't use them if I were you —they spread athlete's foot through the bibliography. I limit myself to about half a dozen which I think are useful. You may think others to be useful—therefore, I am sharing with you a comprehensive list of these devices which I found over a period of many years. For such a list, *v.i.:*

ad fin.—at the end (*ad finem*)
ad inf.—to infinity (*ad infinitum*)
ad init.—at the beginning (*ad initum*)
ad int.—meanwhile (*ad interim*)
ad loc.—to this passage (*ad hunc locum*)
aet.—aged (*aetatis*)
ca. or *c.*—about (*circa*)
cf.—confer (meaning compare) (*conferre*)
c.p.—compare
e.g.—an example (*exempli gratia*)
et al.—and elsewhere (*et alibi*)
et al.—and others (*et alii*)
et seq.—and the following (*et sequens*)
et sqq.—and those following (plural) (*et sequentes* or *et sequentia*)

f. or *ff.*—following pages (or *folios*)
fn.—footnote
i.a.—among others (*inter alia*)
i.e.—that is (*id est*)
i.q.—the same as (*idem quod*)
ibid.—same place (*ibidem*)
id.—same man (*idem*)
idem.—may be same as *ibid.*, or *id.*, or same as before
l.l.—in the place quoted (*loco laudato*)
l. or *ll.*—line or lines
loc. cit.—in the place quoted or cited (*loco citato*)
ms. or *mss.*—manuscript or manuscripts
n.—note
N.B.—mark well (*nota bene*)
n.d.—not dated
n.p.—no publisher given
n.s.—new series
o.p.—out of print
op. cit.—in the work quoted or cited (*opus* [*opere*] *citato*)
pp.—pages (or privately printed)
psm.—here and there—occasionally (*passim*)
q.v.—which see (*quod vide*)
seq.—following (*sequentia*)
sqq.—the following ones (*et sequentes*)
ss.—sections
sic—intentionally so written
s.v.—under the word (*sub verbo*)
s.v.—under the title (*sub voce*)
tr.—translation
u.s.—as above (*ut supra*)
v.—see (vide)
v.—against (versus)
v.i.—see below (*vide infra*)
v.l.—a variant reading (*varia lectio*)
vv.ll.—(plural of above)
v.s.—see above (*vide supra*)
viz—to wit, namely (*videlicet*)

ON SOME WORDS

Many scientific authors, familiar with though not thoroughly comfortable in their language, handle it like the *noveau riche* handle jewelry or other recently acquired goodies: they overdress their writing. They do it by stilted sentences or by the use of presumably fancy words which, misplaced, become monstrosities. It is said that one of the reasons for this phenomenon is that scientists are trained rather than educated. While that may be largely true, we believe that this kind of *writing disease,* more true to medical and other scientific writing, is based on the idea that it confers upon such writers the status of scholars.

Perhaps it is such a dubious belief that writing disease raises status (though it is my belief that it confers infamy) which caused an author to recommend the use of a *monocular occlusion* —when he meant an eyepatch.

Another author gravely informs his reader that a given patient in the case he describes has a *trend to dextrous laterality*—meaning that he, the patient, was righthanded.

Another author speculates on the cause of and discusses the treatment of a *languid disorder.* Unfortunately, the author did not quite realize that the condition was contagious and that the reader may react with the very symptoms of the languid disorder which the author described, namely, fatigue and boredom: the author meant fatigue and boredom when he overdressed them as a *languid disorder.*

Other authors are more compassionate—they use gloriously simple words—which, unfortunately, are distributed into a matrix of diffusion. For example, in an article on oral contraceptives —*the pill*—the author refers to the attitude to *the pill* on the part of Catholic converts. One readily assumes that he refers to non-Catholics who had converted to Catholicism. However, in the context of the article this assumption becomes doubtful, for it reads just as readily as applying to converts *to* Catholicism as to converts *from* Catholicism. Unfortunately, the reader is left without the benefit of the information which the author intended to impart—because he, the author, (a) enshrined it in ambiguity and (b) did not make his meaning clear by defining his subject.

It is the summary, however, which often has the lowest caloric value for the effort expended in reading. It is well known that the summary of an article is often read first to determine if the investment of time in reading the article is warranted. For example, when one meets a sentence such as *The reasons for so-and-so were outlined,* one has drawn a blank. It takes only little more space and it is vastly more informative to summarize that *The reasons for so-and-so reside in the failure of, say, the metabolic conversion of A to B.*

ON PHRASES

Medical writing essentially does not differ from other writing. The objective of all writing is to impart to the reader by symbols called words what the author wishes to convey.

The phrase *it is obvious* is met quite frequently, usually in the form of *the meaning of these results is obvious.* But if the matter is so obvious, it is pointless to mention it. However, the probability is that the matter is not obvious, especially to the nonspecialist. We must not forget that more of writing of medical and other scientific matters is read by people who are *not* specialists in the given subject. *One simple reason is that there are more nonspecialists than specialists in any given area.*

Matter assumed to be obvious may not be obvious by reason of the following: the obviousness may be based on knowledge which has changed, as the recent change in concept that diabetes is due to a deficiency of insulin. Another example: the conclusion drawn may be obvious to the writer, but a reader may see more than one possible conclusion; hence, what is meant may not be obvious to him.

Another phrase is *see chapter. . . .* One finds such references in many texts. But to find, say, chapter nine or any other chapter, it is necessary to go back to the table of contents or to leaf through the book. Having found the chapter, it is at times necessary to look through most of the chapter to find the point to which the text refers. It is so much better to say *see page. . . .*

ON TITLES

The first words of any article are invariably those of the title. Even if the reader first turns to the summary and conclusions to decide if an article is worth his time, he will have first read the title.

For that reason the title should have two attributes: It should *clearly* and *reasonably definitely* express its point. Clarity and definiteness in the title of an article are a help to the reader as well as to the indexer or abstractor. For example, a title such as "The Nature of Sleep Attack" is ambiguous because it is not mutually exclusive—it can mean an attack of anxiety or a heart attack during sleep from which a sleeper awakens. But it can also have a different meaning, namely, a sudden attack of sleep, i.e., narcolepsy.

Other articles are titled merely with the name of a disease, as "Projectile Embolus of the Lung." The reader will ask himself, *What about it? What is a projectile embolus? Is it a description of the disease, its cause, or its therapy?* It turns out to be a four-page article on diagnosis. "Diagnosis of Lung Embolus Caused by a Bullet" would have been more clear and more definite.

The use of a verb often clarifies a title. For example, "Cobalt Heart Disease," though reasonably clear, can be more telling with a title such as "Heart Disease Induced by Cobalt."

Usually a drug or other substance either *does* or *fails to do* something in a disease. A verb introduced into the title of an article clarifies it without unduly lengthening the title. Thus, verbs such as *prevents, induces, enhances, neutralizes,* etc. become quite useful.

Such verbs become increasingly useful in titles of the articles in fields in which there is a divided opinion, as in the anticoagulant field. For example, the title "Anticoagulants After Myocardial Infarction" is so bland as to tell the reader virtually nothing. "Reduced Recurrence of Myocardial Infarction by Anticoagulants" or "Submucous Hemorrhage Induced by Anticoagulants" or even "Ineffectiveness of Anticoagulants" clearly tell in the title the point of the article.

ON JOURNALS

While most articles on medical writing are directed to the writer, few take up the events that occur when a paper finally appears in a journal. We should look into the relationship between journal and reader as it impinges on the usefulness to the reader of a paper that appears in a journal.

No journal editor—no matter how prestigious his journal—can take the haughty position that *his* journal is always saved and bound by the reader, i.e., that papers from his journal are never clipped from it and the remainder of the journal discarded. Fewer journals today are embalmed by the reader! While journal editors are *top dog* to authors who wish to place their papers, the reader is *top dog* to the publication, for journals essentially *compete for the reader's time and storage space.* Realistic journal editors thus accept the fact that if his journal carries worthwhile papers, it will be probably dismembered, and only the papers of interest to a reader will be saved by him.

For those reasons, journals should simplify things for the reader —making it easier for him to clip and file papers appearing in their journals. The greater the number of papers or other items clipped from a given issue, the greater the compliment to the journal. This is a reader's way of saying—"your stuff is worth saving and retrieving."

How can a journal arrange its papers so that they may be clipped whole without invading the entirety of the next paper, which may also be desirable for clipping and filing?

It frequently happens that a reader wishes to clip two or three contiguous papers. Since such papers follow each other without intervening advertising pages, it often happens that a succeeding paper begins on the other side of the page which completes a previous paper. Then, the reader must decide which paper he will clip and save and which he must surrender; he does not necessarily have photoduplication facilities in his office.

Such self-contained papers can be easily arranged in a journal by having papers with an even number of pages follow each other, provided that the first paper, also having an even number of pages, begins on the *right* side of the journal (i.e., on the odd-numbered page). Then each paper—whether two, four, six, or any given even number of pages—becomes self-contained and does not invade a succeeding paper.

Papers which make up an odd number of pages can then follow, provided that the first paper also begins on the odd-numbered page (right side of the journal) and the other side of the last page is used for ancillary matter, i.e., meeting notices, news, or other features which are usually placed in the front of the journal. If we reevaluate our stereotypes, we may find that the last side of a paper which takes up an odd number of pages may produce unexpected assets, for advertisers may vie for these intratextual pages at a premium rate.

Advertising makes the very existence of most periodical journals possible. It is unrealistic to look upon advertising per se as something smacking of contraband or pornography. A journal can refuse advertising copy that is false or even in bad taste. But if such advertising copy is accepted, it should not be hidden when company comes, like the wash a family may be obliged to take in to make ends meet.

One example of what should *not* be done is the arrangement of papers found in the May 1968 issue of a splendid specialty journal. In that issue, the first paper has an odd number of pages—specifically, three pages. The last page of that paper ends on the right side of the journal. And each of the succeeding *six* papers has an even number of pages—hence, each starts on the left side and ends on the right, thus preventing one from clipping two contiguous articles. If the first paper—which had an odd number of pages—had been made the seventh paper, then each of the preceding six papers of even number of papers would have been self-contained.

Other aids to the reader can be easily put into effect. For example, at times, journals publish a paper in two or three installments. While at the end of a given installment the legend *To be continued* is usually given, not always is it noted if a given installment is the first, second, or third part—nor that a given installment is the final one and concludes the paper. The reader often wonders if he has lost the first, a middle, or the final installment. Information on that score gives reassurance that a series is complete.

Other aids to the reader may include a moderately sized, clear font, page number. Have you noticed that in some journals page numbers are considerably smaller than the size of letters in the text? Have you never mistaken a 3 for an 8?

The aim of publication is basically the dissemination of knowledge. If the convenience of the reader is borne in mind, the aim will be enhanced. One method—among others—is to structure a journal so that the reader will be able to clip whole articles even if they are contiguous. And reassure the reader that he did not skip a page—or warn him that he did—by increasing the size of the page numbers!

ON PAY-JOURNALS

It has become stylish to disparage certain free services—as controlled circulation journals. The snob in his fanciful dignity looks down at them but frequently reads them in privacy—much like the proper aunt who would not be caught reading a story that is risqué.

State journals and many other medical and scientific journals for which one pays a subscription fee have this in common with the free or controlled circulation journals: the advertiser. The advertisers absorb the cost of the free journals and defray the cost of those which carry a subscription price.

Since the reduction in advertising creates a deficit too large to absorb, the *Journal of the Indiana State Medical Association* has announced an increase in subscription rates. Other journals have done so too. Literature will become increasingly more expensive for a number of reasons; hence, further increases in subscription rates can be expected.

The opportunity is finally here for the reader who railed against controlled circulation journals to pay his own way. He will finally have the privilege of supporting the journals he reads.

This opportunity should not find him wanting—*but it will.* This means reduced circulation—hence, reduced advertising rates, as the advertising a journal carries is based on circulation. It may also mean a depression in circulation, and advertisers may drop some journals from further consideration. This will further increase costs—and further increases in subscription rates must follow. The information explosion will have fizzled out when it meets a contracting economy. The millennium, probably triggered by Congressional cacophony against advertising expenditures, will have finally come.

ON MULTIPLE SUBMISSIONS

A condition common to all journals is that a paper submitted to it for publication is not simultaneously submitted to other journals.

The custom of exclusive submission of papers for publication has many virtues. It prevents an inadvertent appearance of the identical paper in two or more journals. It allows a journal to build up a backlog. It also enables it to group certain papers—facilitating the easy movement of its backlog. Presumably, the practice also acts as a type of censor, for when a paper is rejected by several publications, the author is to assume that its quality is wanting. The latter is not necessarily the case: a paper may indeed be rejected because of its low caliber. But it may also be rejected for other reasons: (a) the journal may have a huge backlog; (b) the prejudices of the author may not coincide with the prejudices of the editor; and (c) the referees may not have used the best of judgment or probity in their comments, especially when the subject of the paper is quite new, with no precedent.

Ostensibly, the publication of a paper is intended to disseminate a new discovery or finding or otherwise to add to the fund of knowledge. Yet, practically, this is often a secondary consideration. Papers are written and publication is sought by faculty members to increase the number of their publications, which is often taken as a symbol of their standing. Also, papers often serve as a public relations handout.

A published paper is given greater credence than an unpublished report—another compelling and valid need for publication. The increased demands for informational material by the FDA in order to allow the marketing of a drug—or in fact to allow its continuation on the market—should cause an increasing number of papers to be submitted for publication.

But where will these papers be published? The good journals are glutted with papers—and can accept only a small proportion of those offered for publication. Various remedies have been proposed—such as an increased number of journals—and many of these remedies lack realism.

An author's position is becoming increasingly precarious—unless he is a *name*—in which event his papers are sought. Those familiar with the literature are aware of the fact that a *name* and the quality of his reports are not invariably consistent. But *names* die out—places must be found for a new generation of thoughtful authors.

One element, among others, related to the worthiness of a paper is its timeliness. The author is ill-served by a journal to which he submits a paper when the journal takes many months after submission to reject the paper. He then sends the paper to the second journal or to a third journal if it is not accepted by the second one. Each time, three or as many as six months elapse. By the time the paper is published, it may be two years after original submission. The dilatoriness of its referees frequently prevents a journal from advising an author promptly if his paper is accepted for publication or rejected.

The remedy does not necessarily lie in upgrading the quality of the submitted paper as good, though not outstanding papers are also rejected because of the overabundance in the journal's backlog. But a partial remedy may lie in a more expeditious treatment of a paper—promptly informing an author where he stands.

This may be effected by allowing the journals to compete for a paper. This may be done by altering the submission of a paper to one journal at a time—with the long wait imposed upon the author. When a journal will be aware that a paper is submitted simultaneously to two or three journals, it will be competing for a paper it desires and will advise the author within a reasonably short time if his paper has been accepted or rejected. The author, in turn, will probably accept the first notice of acceptance.

Precedents are not necessarily in order to test the adequacy of an idea. Yet, there is a precedent in a related situation: a student sends his application simultaneously to more than one graduate or professional school to which he seeks admission.

Chapter Four

The Moving Finger

CHARLES D. ARING

There arises from a bad and unapt formation of words a wonderful obstruction of the mind.
—FRANCIS BACON

SPOKEN AND WRITTEN COMMUNICATION

WORDS ARE TRICKY; they are powerful instruments, admittedly awkward to handle. Writing is a considerably more difficult way of using words than speech. Communication by sound is an ancient practice which preceded communication in writing. It wasn't too long ago in history that this second step in communicating was taken infrequently, and the populace generally was said to be illiterate. We still run into voluble people whose only ability to communicate in writing is with an *X*. Written communication is the later achievement phylogenetically and ontogenetically. Its neural substrate therefore is not as ingrained and is more readily disordered. Literary effort accordingly requires the greater care. In a sense, writing is a monologue and is

Note: This article represents an expansion of a short note entitled "On Writing for Medical Journals," published in the Editor's Notebook of the *American Journal of Psychiatry, 123*:81–84, July 1966. For permission to rework this material, I have to thank Dr. Francis J. Braceland, the editor of the *American Journal of Psychiatry*.

not subject to the immediate correction of dialogue. Therefore, he who aspires to write must be discerning.

INTELLECT AND EMOTION

Speech and other sound, being the more primitive, have the better access to emotion. It matters more when and how it is said than what is said. Communication in writing usually reflects more nearly intellectual development; it is therefore less reflex. It is a considerably simpler function neurologically to state a message verbally with the usual modicum of perseveration or to belt it out on strings and tom-toms in what often passes for "modern" music.

EXPERIENCE–THE USE OF THE SELF

Regardless of how much one tries, there cannot be communicated what is not known. Untold misery would be avoided if this primary precept were honored. This is reason to foster experience, proper experience. To have lived something usually improves the ability to tell it, more than reading does. Nevertheless, reading is of the essence. Of course, experience has its varieties and vagaries. Several persons are not going to be affected equally by the same happening. Inscrutable genius derives all sorts of impressions from input that touches most of us little, if at all. William James said about this: "Individuality is founded in feeling, and in the recesses of feeling, the darker, blinder strata of character, are the only places in the world in which to catch real fact in the making." Aldous Huxley: "What a gulf between impression and expression! That's our ironic fate—to have Shakespearian feelings and (unless by a billion-to-one chance we happen to be Shakespeare) to talk about them like automobile salesmen or teenagers or college professors. We practice alchemy in reverse—touch gold and it turns to lead; touch the pure lyrics of experience, and they turn into the verbal equivalents of tripe and hogwash."

Experience reflects the uses of the self. One can hardly transmit to another the uses to which the self is put. He can outline what he himself has experienced, how he goes about doing something;

another can then decide whether or not this applies to him and what uses, if any, he wishes to make of it.

SACRED COWS IN WRITING

Another plea for clarity and quality in medical writing may suggest nothing so much as perseveration, but the message can stand repetition. Like freedom, the ideal has no guarantee; it is only constant reworking that fosters it. A standard of excellence to which one can repair in modern letters is the writings of Albert J. Nock. It was during his editorship of *The Freeman* (1920–1924) that Nock enunciated his principles of writing. A young and burgeoning author who was considering *The Freeman* for his productions asked about their policy and if they had any sacred cows. Mr. Nock replied that they certainly had, there were three of them—as untouchable and sacred as the Ark of the Covenant. These were (a) to have a point, (b) to make it out, and (c) to make it out in 18-carat, impeccable, idiomatic English. How charming, how simple, and how difficult!

TOPICS

Medical writing does not require the divine inspiration that is termed *afflatus* in artists or poets. Topics abound in medicine. To have them come tumbling, there is nothing so useful as a healthy curiosity. Samuel Johnson said: "Curiosity is one of the permanent and certain characteristics of a vigorous mind." To illustrate Dr. Johnson's meaning, one need only watch the explorations of a healthy child. Curiosity is likely to regress as one ages.

TECHNIQUE

To make a point requires technique. Technique does not spring forth fully developed as did the wise Athena. Lord Byron's note that easy writing makes damned hard reading still pertains. Technique requires work, and the earlier the practice begins, the better. In our country, unlike Great Britain, little store is set upon the cultivation of rhetoric. We are a practical people, mechanically inclined, and the art and science of using words effectively has been considered somewhat effete. A youngster is more likely to be urged on in sports or social organizations than he is in the cultivation of his language—or any other, for that matter. This barrier is transcended by few Americans, and its effect on the ability to express ideas in writing is ubiquitous.

The amazing natural capacity of the normal brain to sop up a language begins between the second and sixth years; compared with the difficulty encountered later on, it is reminiscent of a sponge, gradually losing capacity to hold water. Most of us missed the prize on the first go-round at home or in school. We did not learn to communicate clearly. I find that the best I was able to do later in compensation was to search out my models consciously. Obviously, this implies disciplined reading and resolute dedication to a fine dictionary. Models do not make up completely for lost opportunity, although I know of no better replacement. My own grammatical competence remains the amateur. I find Lincoln's quotations peculiarly appropriate: "I can never think except with my fingers," and "Punctuation is with me a matter of feeling rather than education." A small point, perhaps idiosyncratic: I do my best writing (or editing) in the early morning.

MODELS

For those who aren't readily put off by his sometimes outrageous statements, I offer Nock as a model. Nock can do much for the style of physicians who write. Reading his last book,[4] *Memoirs of a Superfluous Man,* is a pleasant way of assimilating his sacred cows. Quiller-Couch defined good manners in writing as style. It is regrettable that in general, good manners have gone out of style. In my own writing, I identify with the reader and try to look at what I have written from the standpoint of one or another of my peers conjured up for the occasion.

My physician models are Wilfred Trotter, that expert at phrasing the principles and philosophies of medicine, and his pupil, Sir Francis Walshe. Trotter is readily sampled in his collected papers,[6] and Sir Francis is still writing as vigorously and as beautifully as ever. Nock, Trotter, and Walshe all exhibit exquisitely modulated senses of humor. Lacking humor, man is benighted.

WRITING IN MEDICAL SCHOOL

Better writing could be fostered by schools of medicine. The competences students bring with them to medical school go largely unattended by a medical faculty. Medical students are able and interesting people with individual abilities and interests. Some are inclined musically, others esthetically, electrically, artistically, or religiously; a few even have some literary competence. Ignoring talent suggests that the student is not bringing anything of moment to medicine, whereas absolutely *any experience is grist for the medical mill.* One illustration is the use of the English language. Our students have been required to compose more effectively in high school and college than in medical school. If they have grown up without this discipline and their writing is undisciplined, graduate school is the place to put an end to this neglect! The indifference of medical schools to clear writing has encouraged the profession to foster a thoroughly reprehensible "medicalese."

JARGON

"Medicalese" is a branch of what Bernstein [1] called inside talk, or "officialese," or perhaps better, Washington Choctaw. Jargon may aid communication among members of a sect or union or profession but at the risk of inbreeding. As Bernstein points out, it often goes awry; then jargon becomes "windyfoggery." The problem in addiction to specialized gobbledygook is surely a training deficiency, which practically guarantees inability to express thoughts clearly.

One can supplement for training that has been missed; character deficit is another matter. A scrupulous honesty with oneself—the dedication to see things as they are and not as one wishes them to be—should become second-nature by nurture. This quality cannot be said to be well-established. Bernstein notes "windyfoggery" may come from a wistful desire to make learned sounds or to cover a paucity of information. There are always limitations to knowledge. The healthy practitioner should be moved to acknowledge openly what he honestly doesn't know. When internal security or knowledge is below par, a wordy obfuscation often results. I advocate a look behind the camouflage as an exercise in straightforwardness.

Within a group there always develops a private kind of language. In the teenager, enmeshed in confusions about who he is and other insecurities, a mystic bond is forged with peers in an odd and angular patois. This kind of communication takes temporary precedence, but there comes a time in life when this tendency should be renounced.

REWORKING

Reviewing what I have written in my early drafts, I am amazed at the insipid and inadequate phrasing—in short, failure of expression. Most of us must rely on the onerous chore of reworking. We have to reach within ourselves without fear or anxiety to find what it is we want to say and to whom. We must correct and correct until every statement says what is meant to its intended reader. Thackeray said: "The only good writing is re-writing." One strives for that perfection where rereading a decade or so later suggests little change. It is the rare genius, like Mozart or Schubert, who can work out a line in his mind, then set it down and leave it. Everything must be rewritten over and over and over and in half the number of words, which takes twice as long, to paraphrase Garland,[3] and in Nock's 18-carat, impeccable, idiomatic English, untainted by "medicalese."

GOOD MANNERS

The writer should consider that he is holding a dialogue in which he must speak ever so much more clearly than he does in conversation because he cannot hear his interlocutor. He must develop good manners in writing; I have heard about an editor who said: "I never read beyond the first cliché." Most medical editors are willing to hurdle clichés in their attempt to find whether the writer has a point. This gives me the opportunity to indict a few medical examples: definitive, in regard to, parameter, status (which means position in society), case (for patient), male (for man), passed away, sacrificed, denies (who's accusing?), autopsy (for necropsy), visualize (which means to form a mental picture of), space-occupying (what doesn't?), marked, very, or any superlative. These are remindful of *Adventures in Wonderland* where "Alice had not the slightest idea what latitude was, or longitude either, but she thought they were nice grand words to say." What is euphemistically termed *the literature* might be reduced to manageable proportions by ruthless exclusion of articles laced with clichés, to say nothing about papers based on insignificant or inconclusive statistics.

CONTENT VERSUS FORM

In scientific writing, content versus form is treated often enough as dichotomous. An amusing essay by Wilson,[7] entitled "Better Written Journal Papers—Who Wants Them?," is concerned with the problem. Editors of scientific publications generally are more intent on content. But Dalessio[2] describes the fallacy of cutting too fine a line, and he illustrates delightfully by editing a few excerpts from classical poetry.

ORIGINAL	OFFICIAL REVISED VERSION
Andrew Marvell "To His Mistress"	
But at my back I always hear *Time's wingéd chariot hurrying near;*	I am aware that Time is passing.
Percy Bysshe Shelley "To a Skylark"	
Hail to thee, blithe spirit!	Hello, bird.
Leigh Hunt "Abou Ben Adhem"	
Abou Ben Adhem (may his tribe increase!) *Awoke one night from a dream of peace,* *And saw within the moonlight in his room,* *Making it rich, and like a lily in bloom* *An angel writing in a book of gold:*	Mr. Adhem awakened Hallucinating.

I don't see why competence in one area need be accompanied by incompetence in another. There is, though, a curious human tendency to consign the broadly competent expert to a field other than one's own, no doubt some indication of the consigner's anxieties.

I am dedicated to the propositions (a) that the literate scientist is possible and (b) that there is an essential unity in science and literature. Surely, as Elizabeth Sewell[5] said, poetry puts language to full use as a means of thought, exploration, and discovery. For example, poets and writers enunciated the tenets of the schools of psychology and psychiatry before these disciplines were born. Victor Hugo saw poetry as an instrument of research into the enigmas of the mind and nature. René Dubos calls the poet the conscience of humanity, noting that poets, novelists, and artists commonly anticipate what is to be achieved one or two generations later by technological and social means. Aristotle's pronouncement bears: "The poets have the advantage of expressing the universal; the specialist expresses only the particular."

A REASON TO WRITE

Without the dedication and kindness of my chiefs and of senior physicians and editors, I might have been denied the considerable pleasure of writing. Writing affords the opportunity to balance inner urges and imposed controls in a kind of mastery of the self. If it is possible, it represents a function not to be denied. Youth trying always deserves respect. Ideally, editorial irritation should be reserved for those who show little willingness to improve, who remain above the development of Pascal's "wise ignorance which recognized itself." I have derived no better sacred cows than my model, Albert J. Nock: to have a point, to make it out, and to make it out in 18-carat, impeccable, idiomatic English; but these thoughts on the *how* of it may be useful.

THERE IS NOTHING NEW UNDER THE SUN

It is fitting to close with a quotation from the great John Locke. This philosopher, who was also a physician, obviously was troubled by the jargon and prolixities abroad in the seventeenth century, when he said: "Vague and insignificant forms of speech and abuse of language have so long passed for mysteries of science, and hard or misapplied words, with little or no meaning have been . . . mistaken for deep learning. They are but covers of ignorance and hindrance of true knowledge."

References

1. Bernstein, T. M.: *The Careful Writer. A Modern Guide to English Usage.* New York, Atheneum Publishers, 1965, p. 487.
2. Dalessio, D. J.: Grace and Merriment in Medical Writing, *Medical Opinion and Review, 3:*60–62, July 1967.
3. Garland, J.: The Art of Communication. *International Records of Medicine, 169:*703–709, 1956.
4. Nock, A. J.: *Memoirs of a Superfluous Man.* Chicago, Regnery, 1964, p. 326.
5. Sewell, E.: *The Orphic Voice.* New Haven, Yale University Press, 1960 p. 463.
6. Trotter, W.: *The Collected Papers of Wilfred Trotter.* London and New York, Oxford University Press, 1941. p. 194.
7. Wilson, J. H., Jr.: Better Written Papers—Who Wants Them? *Science, 165:*986–987, September 5, 1969.

Chapter Five

The Art of Writing Papers

WALTER C. ALVAREZ

OFTEN WHEN I start to write a paper, there comes to my mind a well-remembered scene which occurred late one evening some forty years ago, when I went to say goodnight to my overworked general practitioner father. It was shortly after 10 P.M. when he came in from what he hoped was his last call for the night. On going into his room, I saw him sitting up in bed with several medical journals spread about him. I can never forget what he said:

> Oh, Walter, why don't they make the articles short for physicians like me, who so want to keep up with medical progress but who have, at the end of the day, only half an hour or so in which to read? Also, why won't they use simpler English? Tonight I am so tired that I cannot easily read complicated sentences. Perhaps on Sunday afternoon, when I am rested, I will be able to read a badly-written text, full of puzzling words, like parameter and paradigm, but tonight I just can't face such prose.

Another experience of long ago gave me another important thought about writing. A young woman physiologist said to me that after a year's research, her paper had twice been sent back by editors. Would I please tell her what was wrong with it? When I tried to read it, it was so badly written that I could not even guess what she had done or what she had found. After much questioning, I still could not get a clear idea of what she had done. Finally, she said, "Never mind; I can't be bothered to rewrite it. *I write only to please myself anyway.*" She left, and I never saw her again. What impressed me about her statement was that always when a man writes, he should be thinking of his audience. Is it a lay group, an audience of practicing physicians, or one of research chemists? Obviously, what will please and instruct one group will only bore or go over the heads of another. Many an article, I believe, sent to a clinical journal should have been sent to a research publication.

Many a time in my many years of preparing lectures, I have had to puzzle over what phase of a subject might possibly hold the interest of all of *four* groups. Without fail, at the final evening banquet of some big association of specialists, I see before me a diverse audience of practicing physicians, wives, a scattering of laymen, plus a group of eminent research men.

Every man who aspires to write would do well to try to create prose that will interest and please a few thousand readers to the extent that they will read all of his article but more, will want to read the next several articles written by him. For myself, there are a few physicians in this country whose papers and books I will stop to read. Why? Because through the years their writings have always given me not only much useful information but pleasure and mental stimulation.

How does one acquire skill in writing? I am sorry to say my impression is strong that a really good writer *inherits* most of his ability. I am almost convinced of this because of the phenomenon of writing ability that keeps turning up in two or three generations of certain families, like the Huxleys. Another reason why I think a gift for skillful writing is inborn is that I have known so many able and well-educated men who did not have the art and worse, could never learn it. Perhaps heredity has something to do with the curious fact that I write a syndicated newspaper column; my son Robert writes a monthly newsletter full of ideas for executives, and my daughter Gladys writes a weekly newsletter for her church.

A curious and sad fact is that although I have written day after day for sixty-three years, the task of "boiling down," polishing, and rearranging what I have written has never grown easier. One would think that such editorial skill would come with years of experience, but I see no sign of it. Today, the work seems just as difficult as when I wrote and published my first medical paper in 1906, as an intern. My only comfort is that one of my literary heroes, the brilliant Robert Louis Stevenson, once said in his later years that with the passage of time, writing became no easier for him; he still had to rewrite many times.

When friends ask "From whom did you get your style?" my answer has been that I never tried to copy anyone. I have always loved Osler's writings, but I have never attempted to write as he did, with many interesting quotations from the ancients and others. Obviously, if a man is to write well enough to interest and instruct his readers, he must be very well-read in his field; he should be a master of his subject; he should be up-to-date, and—this is the important point—he should take pleasure in telling of the excellent but perhaps overlooked work of able men who preceded him in his field. To do this is to be honest and kind and helpful to one's antecedents and readers.

Often I have found it helpful to try a paper out on my wife and my secretaries to see if they liked and could understand what I had written. And often they have helped with excellent criticisms and suggestions. Many a time my wife will note that a sentence which I thought could have only one meaning really could convey another impression. Then, of course, it had to be rewritten. Often a secretary will make the valid suggestion that I add a few words to define a rare term.

During my many years as an editor, when I had to study papers sent for publication, I often disapproved of those with a long introduction or others with one or two introductory pages describing a chemical technic used in the research. Such prologues would probably discourage many readers from tackling the article. Often I wrote to the author, suggesting that he delete the lengthy introduction and put the description of his research technic at the end of his paper, where it could be studied by those few who would wish to repeat his experiments. Many years ago I was given a good lesson by a writer of advertising copy. He said, "In our game we try to grab the interest of people with the first sentence, and then, we try desperately, to hang onto that interest."

Another lesson I learned as an editor selecting articles for publication was that when a man sends an article about some old and much-worked-over subject (such as gastric analysis), he should anticipate that the editor will probably groan and ask, "What on earth can anyone write on *that* topic that will be of interest?" Hence, if I were now writing on, let us say, abdominal pain, I would begin, "Strange to say, there is a fairly common type of abdominal pain which is rarely diagnosed correctly," and I would hope the editor would then be sufficiently intrigued to read on to see what I had to say. And perhaps a few thousand physicians would also stop to look and read.

Incidentally, the present-day custom of putting an abstract of an article at the top and not at the end of an article is ideal. So many thousands of us busy doctors have time only to read an abstract. Also, because so many will read only the abstract, the wise author will see to it that it is written with the greatest care.

A good idea sometimes is to put a finished manuscript aside for a month or two or more. Then, when I pick it up again, I can rewrite it as ruthlessly as if I were correcting some other man's paper.

Incidentally, the wise writer should spend much time devising an attractive and very short title for his paper. As we all know, a good title can sometimes make a good book into a best seller. Also, the writer would do well to remember that it is pertinent to entitle his paper in a manner to facilitate its retrieval in annual literature indexes. For example, many years ago when Jacobi discovered the interesting reverse peristalsis in the right side of the colon, instead of providing it with a suitable title, he buried his discovery in an article on poisoning with colchicum.

A thoughtful writer, I think, will avoid complex tables because so few readers will study them. Sometimes, data could be illustrated better in a graph; then I would hope that the writer would identify his ordinates and abscissas so that the readers could quickly understand what the graph meant.

Many of the case reports I have seen could be greatly shortened; findings of no significance should be omitted. Often I have seen a long necropsy report with dozens of pointless details which should have been deleted. When a necropsy showed that the man died of a carcinoma of the pancreas, who wants to know dozens of minor details?

One thing I dislike about some writers is their fondness for writing *emesis* for vomiting and *singultus* for hiccuping.

Finally, I would suggest that more writers fill their articles with facts of observation and devote less space to theorizing and speculation. Think how wonderful it would have been if the old writers in medicine had filled their books with exact descriptions of syndromes, such as angina pectoris, gallstone colic, multiple sclerosis, and gastric crises of tabes. We would revere them ever so much more than we do as we read of their curious theories of disease etiology such as moist or dry, the four humours, or demoniac possession.

Chapter Six

Ruminations on the Physician as a Writer

WILLIAM B. BEAN

I HAVE no expectation that another essay or a sermon, lecture, or catalogue of caveats for writers will do any good. Hundreds of books on how to write are readily available. Some are written well. Some are written not so well, and some have a curiously unpleasant knack of illustrating the very faults they decry. I allowed myself to be cajoled into writing this dirge ostensibly to help those who want to be helped, but probably more because I was flattered to be asked.

A more fruitful effort might have been to study the reasons for neglect of the ample body of books and papers which gives useful instruction in good writing. The sorry state of writing seen in so many medical journals today can be looked upon as a symptom of the ascendancy of technology and techniques which everywhere is overwhelming us in torrents of pollution. Our air is filled with acrid smog, our rivers with sewage and industrial wastes, and our food with toxic residues. By a universal breach of the law of parsimony, our medical journals similarly are filled with technical outpourings of barely literate scientists and medical men. Too often the untutored but enthusiastic physician, coyly succumbing to the urge to commit something to writing, only excretes more sewage into the journalistic *Cloaca Maxima.* The repository for these excretions is dignified by one of the great euphemisms of all time under the term *the literature.*

The real problem of confronting those who are concerned with the bleak absence of style, form, and excellence from medical writing surely is not a dearth of information about how to improve things. The real question is *Why do people fail to read, mark, learn, and assimilate all the readily available material?* Any medical or scientific person who writes should have ready access to and use several kinds of helpful books. Everybody needs dictionaries, grammars, and collections of synonyms, jargon, and usage. In addition, there are many very fine manuals, technical books, and guides to good writing. A third collection is no less essential for those who wish to pursue writing to the point of real excellence and a personal style. This is a personal selection of one's favorite from the many classical books which may be studied for style, for method, and for process, as well as for content. We must learn how the best writers manage a felicitous interaction of matter and manner permeated with feeling, sense, and interest to produce classical literature. In confronting books, one may nibble or browse or graze or ruminate after the manner of cattle. They eat and then chew their cud. From very unpromising raw material their own digesting and fermenting vats create a rich, sustaining end product which is enhanced by the vigorous action of biosynthesis.

English idiom and idiomatic use are so hard to learn that the foreigner almost despairs of mastering English. In varying degrees this is true of any person with any foreign language. Those who have been brought up where language is respected and revered gain sufficient mastery from innumerable corrections and from unconscious assimilation. Instruction in idiomatic expression is superfluous. For these fortunate ones it is automatic. When questioned, he may not know exactly what rule governs his correct usage. He finds, as did Moliere's character, that he'd been speaking *prose* all along. The real difficulty which most of us have when we move from the spoken language, which is commonly correct and clear enough, to the written language is that we put on the formal gear of obscurantism and camouflage. Just let the physician approach a typewriter or take up a pen and he dons therewith a mask of obscurity. A stilted and unnatural jargon-filled paper is the demoralizing end product.

Reading aloud what one has written brings things back into the more natural context of conversation. It is a chastening but useful practice. While experts suggest that writing a speech and writing an essay are two different things, almost any essay will be improved by removing acerbities and banalities which are revealed when it is read aloud, particularly by someone not the writer. Good writing should be tonally, rhythmically, and intellectually satisfying as it is heard by the spoken voice. It is discouraging to hear one's own words read aloud for criticism. At least it prepares one for the trauma experienced when our self-confident and self-comforting extemporaneous remarks are captured on tape and then transcribed. It may produce an effect like a parody on some of Eisenhower's less coherent press conferences. At best, this reminds every writer that he owes a greater number of courtesies to his reader and will not be forgiven indefinitely if he forgets them.

Perhaps this homily can begin by concentrating on examples of bad writing I have culled from sundry manuscripts.

Let us begin our exercise by assuming that a doctor has been asked to write a short paper on a bird and an animal. His "scientific" paper begins:

> The author deemed that this assignment should be envisaged and structured before it was implemented by us. The avian creature which it appears is to be written about by us as part of the overall dialogue is a nocturnal, night-flying dark adapted feathered creature of prey of the family of *Strigiformes.* This denizen of the woods does not possess measurable visual capacity of any really significant degree when it is measured by measuring it during the hours of daylight. During the nocturnal period, the owl has been described as being "blind as a bat"—an obvious mistake.
>
> Since we have not been basically informed with guidelines from a high level nor have we been exposed to a data about the members of the order of *Strigiformes,* it is apparent that we should begin to proceed to initiate the strategies of our dialogue on the creature which has been chosen by us as the subject for rendition of the more extended portion of our so-called essay. Whether it is knowledgeable or disadvantaged is not known to us. The cow has been chosen by us as our key subject for high level writing. This animal has been localized in the class of *Mammalia* for the reason that it is a vertebrate which feeds the young from externally appended organs of lactation. The cow may be considered as a modified cube,

roughly a six-sided mammal, with its external aspects, planes, and surfaces superior, inferior, anterior, posterior, dexter, and sinister. Articulated to the superior-posterior region of the mammal's anatomy is the nonprehensile tail which it is of interest to say has many long cow-tail-hairs coming from the terminal extremity which constitutes the end of this beast's nonvestigial caudal appendage. With this it decimates flies, thus mitigating against their falling into the lacteal fluid. This organ makes the former more likely than the latter, although formerly the latter was less unlikely than the former was latterly. Cephalad is an organ designated, sited, and suited for hanging the horns on, a mammalian trophy room rather than a mark of infidelity. As an afterthought, it ought to be recalled by us that the oral machinery must be insured of a place to be ensconced in order to be appropriately positioned, placed, and put environmentally. The horns are the weapons which it is said of, "never has so much been done with so little to so many," or something like that. The mouth is present as an organ with which the mooing is produced by the rapid vibration of the mechanically activated and resonating vocal cords.

In the posterior-inferior part of the specimen, a non Caucasian, nonwhite, nonmale (i.e. female) is hung the udder or the organ by which the cow is recognized as being a natural member of the mammal family. The design of the pendent processes protruding from the udder is recognized as being related to the method of milk produced and the selfsame aforesaid milk being made ready for delivery when activated by a milkmaid's hands, a calf's mouth, or a vacuum pump. Milk might be defined as nothing but unprocessed cheese, with the fluid "gang aft a whey."

The never ending substantive production of substantive milk may be looked upon as a substantive method of keeping unprocessed substantive grass from having its substance wasted. The usage of pasturage is great, grasswise. In the bovine creature the removal of milk leaves a vacuum into which grass is placed prior to cud chewing, digestion, assimilation, and milk making. The purpose of this is to often, if not continually, help make milk made. But how? By what process? In what manner? and by what device the procedure is accomplished is, it might have been said by us, a bovine dialogue for high-level personnel. It works well. It fails. Anymore, it requires a follow-up. Presently, feel free to study bovine conditions for your answer.

The methodology by which the bovine mammal is found to have been an agent in having lacteal fluids produced is direct proof of overall proportions. It is not all that important (how much?), it is not that milk (what?), it is not that way (which?), it is not that complicated (how much?). The female of the bovine mammal has much sense of smell but no smell of sense. The stimulus impinging on the olfactory organ enables one to scent its presence at a marked, large, great, and considerable separation from the beast which is the source and site of production.

Failure of substantial attenuation of the malodorous scent, smell, stink, and stench as far as a multitude of cases of modern scientific and critical as well as careful research is said to seem to have gone, mitigates against understanding. This is the alleged reason not unfresh, unsubstantial vapors exist far away from the urban areas, ghettos, and suburban sprawls (i.e. the country). The masculine member of the cow family, no cow, is said to present signs of being an ox (*e.g.; sotto voce; dolce far niente*—a bull). The bull is a mammal only by courtesy and a play on words. Grass eaten by the cow is eaten twice or many times so that a little goes a long way. Be careful in cow pastures. Hunger contractions, spasms, pangs of pains are considered to be activating mechanisms to initiate the neuro-musculo-servo-pneumo-audio-bellow activity, so-called mooing. But it doesn't all sound all that loud. It hears good. When a cow is full it is contented. No sounds are made by the cow to impinge on our aural organs. In short, there is no noise soundwise.

Critique

The introduction demonstrates almost casual indifference to the subject. Let us take our examples bit by bit to see how to clear up the mess. How should we treat the assigned topic? The person who really wants to write clearly must be active and write by attacking the problem directly. Now, to go through the example word by word, a painful process but necessary for our lesson.

When one person is writing, and it is rare for two to hold the pen simultaneously, he can use the pompous wallflower words *the author*. But *the author* are bloomer words recalling a spurious modesty never fooling anyone and in our miniminded and miniskirted time are being overcorrected by the Grand Canyon view of the femoral triangle. Mock modesty is bad; modesty, a virtue, is declining but improves writing by making it simple. Unless one is of such corpulent dimensions that he is recognized as a group, a true collective noun, or harbors tapeworms or nits and thus is plural *de facto* or wants to be self-important, avoid *we*. Editors may *we* us if they like. Occasionally *we* makes stale discourse lively. But when one person is identified as writing or caught speaking, "we" is affected.

Deemed

If you catch anyone *deeming* anything, it is best to get out of range.

Envisaged

If this thought really needs to be put in, use *seen, looked at,* or *thought of.*

Structured

Structure as a lame verb has helped to decompose the language. Possibly it is an intrusion from the engineers, though more likely it came from bureaucrats. When you encounter the word *structured* in a document or see an old edifice *edificing* something, hold your hands over your head and count three. Plaster may be coming down from the decaying intellectual ceiling.

Implement

Since World War II got tooled up, almost nothing gets done. It gets *implemented. Implement* is a grandiose word for tool. Wherever you see the word *implement,* substitute *shovel.* This gives the proper nuance of function.

Avian creature

In a textbook of zoology, or indeed one dealing with birds in an aviary, this may pass, but it does not simplify things. It is a throwback or residual trace of the *Comestock load* (I mean load), a bowdlerizing blush which designated a bull as a gentleman cow, to Mencken's loud howls of delight.

It appears

If one could expunge *it seems, it appears, it is likely,* and *it is apparent* from all writing by insecure people, a million years of reading time would be saved.

The great insecurity of most who write of medicine and science is demonstrated by the weakening influence of the passive voice. Instead of saying "I will write," they say "It will be written by me." Editors now wearily accept the melancholy awkwardness of the passive which obscures, delays, and distends the passage.

Overall

Overalls, an important part of the gear of a farmer, are best left out of writing and speech. Wherever you see the word *overall,* strike it out. I have encountered *overall* many hundred times. I always remove it. I have yet to find an example where striking it out did not send the writing in the direction of clarity and away from confusion. In clear writing each word is important. Study every word. Dissect modifiers. Destroy the useless ones.

Here is a great bit of advice to the person who wishes to use a modifier. When you want to modify, judge what happens if you use the antithesis, or opposite. Is it clearer? Or different? What happens if you leave it out entirely? When you have an uncontrollable urge to say *overall,* substitute *overnone,* or even *undernone.* It livens up a bleak sentence.

Dialogue

The word *dialogue* is used mostly by masters of monologue. Often it is monotone. *Dialogue* occasionally refers to an exchange of ideas which might occur in a discussion, debate, argument, or a donnybrook which had progressed into a street fight. It used to be a good word, but it has had its utility and virility abraded away by our abuse.

Night-flying feathered creatures of prey, the family of Strigiformes

This sort of nonsense is simply the way doctors and scientists often write when they think no one is watching. This pseudoelegant *package* consists of a superfluous superfluity of pleonastic and tautological redundancy. In short, it is an example of linguistic supererogation. This is the way deep-lunged-large-vital-capacitied-windjammers make out when they want to say owl. It is as bad as *This denizen of the woods. Measurable visual capacity* is merely another long way around. So is *of any really significant degree,* and the same goes for *during the hours of daylight.* Such elliptical comments should make us wince at so much *medical* writing.

During the nocturnal period

This genteel obliquity Ernest Gowers calls puddery. Then the passive again.

Blind as a bat

One can use a cliché as his own or put it in quotes as a kind of protective denial. We would die without clichés. But they are not brought out for our favorite guests.

This laborious introduction to the writing of a simple scientific essay was handled much better by a child of ten when requested to write an essay on an animal and a bird. The first paragraph went as follows: "The bird that I am going to write about is the owl. The owl cannot see at all by day and at night is blind as a bat." This is all that is needed.

Have not been basically informed

Basically is unnecessary. It makes a high level seem even more awkward than necessary, intruding into the middle of a compound verb. Often such intrusion is not noticed. It may sound natural. But here it is bad.

High level

Level is a word which has gotten out of hand. It is something dear to the hearts of bureaucrats and sociologists. About one time out of ten it means something.

Been exposed

Awkward and passive.

A data

The language is full of hundreds of words which have had their original meaning ground off, their derivation forgotten. They may become marvelous instruments of fertile and sometimes poetic expression. The transition in use and meaning may take a couple of years, a couple of decades, a generation or two, or longer. Some do not make the grade, for example, the word *ain't,* which serves a very useful purpose for the awkward *am I not. Data* as a plural is fading away. Misuse of *data* does not separate the high from the low IQs but separates those who are word blind and deaf from those who are perceptive. But anyone trying to enforce rules for a word's acceptance or rejection should study Old King Canute's injunction to the naughty tide which kept wetting his feet.

There is something wonderfully reassuring about making errors in writing or pronunciation—if enough people are wrong often enough, wrong becomes right. Use establishes custom, precedent becomes law. The matter is not so much clarity as the fact that the *nouveaux,* whether in terms of language or money, rarely have taste. In medical and scientific writing, if one wishes to model his language on the truly expert, he will attend to such picayune matters as making subject and predicate agree, even if he has to go a little beyond the funny papers for his inspiration.

A member of the Strigiformes *family*

The sesquipedalian stridor again. Puddery is for the insecure, the idle, or those paid by the word.

We should begin to proceed to initiate

See *Night-flying feathered creatures of prey, the family of* Strigiformes.

Discourse

See *Dialogue.*

Creature which

See first paragraph of Critique.

Has been chosen by us

See *It appears.*

For rendition as

See *Have Not Been Basically Informed.* A so-called essay.

Ours

See second paragraph of Critique.

So called

Unnecessary.

Essay

A proud word for a paper but sometimes a good one.

Has been chosen

See *It appears.*

Key subject

Poor word choice.

This animal

A dainty substitute for the cow.

Localized

It may be better to say *localized* than the overused *place* for *put.* Almost no one now can bear to use the simple word *put.* Everything is *placed* these days. I am against it.

For the reason that

An elliptical statement for *because.*

A Vertebrate

This is clear enough but a little fancy.

Externally appended organs of lactation

Many people are made uneasy or perhaps get stimulated and overexcited by the whole notion of breasts, udders, mammals, and lactation. This is so much so that young women with an urge to flap themselves about as go-go girls, if not particularly well endowed by nature, may have whatever they have filled up by plastic bubbles, a source of considerable scientific interest and a new variety of lesion.

An Aside on Busts

A funny custom in the West
Disturbs the woman with flat breast,
So Symmers thought up silicone
To shape them like a hilly cone.
I think this makes girls feel less cowed
When they compete with more endowed
Disporters flaunting natural fonts
In lively topless restaurants.
Oh, far away these girls have drifted
From those who had their face uplifted.
As Symmers, in his Case Reports,
Shows to what length a girl resorts,
For their deficiencies atone
By introducing silicone. It might lead on
to fun and froligue
Improved by someone's "plastic colleague."

"As her bust was small, her fiance persuaded her to allow a plastic colleague to implant a sealed polyethylene bladder behind each breast." It was the impression that in the ordinary wear and tear the deflation might be repaired by going to the filling station as we do for a tire with a slow leak.

Perhaps a few are put off from using the word *udder* by recalling the atrocious pun alleged to be a comment mooed out in a low moan by a dowager cow pursued by a young bull as she miscalculated the height of a barbed wire fence she was trying to leap over. She said "I am udderly ruined." [1]

Modified cube

A cow is pretty hard to describe to someone who has never seen one (purple or not). *Cube* is not such a bad start. It gives one the orthodox six surfaces, perhaps suggesting that the writer is a square. Maybe this really is the very best way to think about a cow. Nonetheless, the terms *superior, interior, anterior, dexter,* and *sinister* for *upper, lower, front, back, right,* and *left* might be thought affectation.

Articulated

A nice, long, juicy word for *fastens to* or *hangs on.*

Superior-posterior region

We get into some pretty unattractive terrain here. Maybe it is clearer than *at the back* or the Aussie *outback.*

The mammal's anatomy

This is like *anatomy, pathology, surgery, astronomy,* and *pediatrics.* Use a long, sonorous rumble for a shorter word. Here *anatomy* means *body, pathology* usually means *lesion, astronomy* often represents the *heavens* or the *stars,* and so on.

Nonprehensile

An incursion in praise of the wisdom of the writer.

It is of interest to say

See *It appears.*

Long cow-tail-hairs coming from the terminal extremity

See *Night-flying feathered creatures of prey, the family of* Strigiformes.

Decimate

Decimate is such a juicy word that people use it when they mean something between *clobbers* and *destroys.* It means reducing by 10 percent, but there is something grand about it, like the word *Mesopotamia* or *apocalypse,* which guarantees it a long life among the dullards.

Mitigate

It is curious that while *mitigate* is often used for *militate,* I do not remember seeing it the other way around. *Mitigate* means to lessen or soothe or soften, and *militate* has the proper sound and fury of waging war or opposing mightily. It is rarely needed in current prose but chosen often with flamboyant ignorance. Watch it.

Them

Should be *their.*

Lacteal fluid

Genteel obfuscation.

Former and latter

Whenever you see *former* and *latter,* you know the writer is too lazy to write clearly enough not to send you back a few words, a sentence, a paragraph, or a page to see what he is trying to say. Generally, it is not worth going back for.

Cephalad is an organ

Okay in a highly technical paper on anatomy or neurology but block it in simple prose. Here we have the passive voice, tautology, and a coyness not altogether fresh. Beware of a writer's desire to be witty unless it helps with the exposition. It is a matter of taste, and good taste has gone from literature these days when everyone has forgotten the antique wisdom that children should be obscene and not heard.

Horns or weapons

Fancy.

Never has so much

A misapplied misquotation.

Is present

Every now and then I hear someone describing something in medicine by saying *the presence of pain was present, or was absent.* This fairly well gathers up a nest of errors.

Organ with which the mooing is produced

Passive, oblique.

Rapid vibration of the mechanically activated vocal cords

Fancy.

Specimen

Unnecessary synonym.

Non-Caucasian

If one could eliminate the negative complexes and the offensive incursions of -ise, -ize, and -wise at the end of words, writing would be clearer and simpler. In my whole life I have met only two people I have recognized as coming from the Caucasus. I marvel at the deployment of Caucasian as a synonym for white.

Male and female

Fine for dealing with creatures like cows and bulls but not for a single person among our fellows, our patients, and colleagues whom we would not introduce at a cocktail party, at least while sober, as a *male* or a *female.* After all, at a time when sex in adolescents was becoming obscured by pants and cheerfully flowing hair,

The mini-skirt in any stance
solved the problem at a glance.

We should concede to present wishes and use *Black* for *Negro,* which reverses the efforts of more than a hundred years. Suddenly it has become nearly universal.

Pendent processes protruding

Alliteration is well and good, but the word *teat* is simpler.

Being produced

See *It appears.*

Selfsame or foresaid

This is usually an unnecessary intrusion from legal documents. Such words rarely clarify. It is the same sort of tic, engendered of insecurity, which fills a paper with *as was mentioned by us prior to now,* or *as will be discussed in a subsequent page.* Also, *above* or *below* are rarely needed, and they may be made inaccurate if the printer breaks a page in the wrong place, making up down and vice versa.

Delivery

An obstetrical or post office word.

Activated by

Clear but long.

Unprocessed cheese

Milk is indeed unprocessed cheese. So is a tree unprocessed lumber. But *milk* is simpler.

"Gang aft a whey"

A quote, a pun, or a misquote are all right but should be used sparingly. Unless one has complete control, they are intrusions. In conversation, puns offend those who did not think of them because of their slower association machinery. But use such decorations sparingly, like good perfume.

Substantive

What was said previously about *overall* might be said about *substantive.* Either something is *substantive* or it is not. If it is not, forget about it. Do not waste time. Never mention it. Certainly it is not worth writing a paper about or describing. I am not eager to have anybody tell me about subjects they believe have no substance. This egregious tautology should be stricken from every sentence in every paper and every conversation. Forget it. If you see it or hear it, suspect the person who has used it. Or at least frown.

Usage

Terms like *usage* for *use, dosage* for *dose,* and *methodology* for *method* make a writer seem a little bit more important—but only to himself.

"Milk leaves"

Not likely to confuse, but words with several meanings may be misread several times before they become clear. This is rare with the spoken word in ordinary talking.

I have given up hope of restoring the word *before. Before* has all but disappeared from the language. Although *prior to* is Latin and ugly, it thrives because people do not think about how they speak or write.

Cud chewing, etc.

Unnecessary perseveration. The stuck-needle syndrome.

To often if not continually help make milk made

It is all right to split infinitives if you know what you are doing, but the long wait for the rest of the verbs makes the sentence Latin or Germanic, with the verb coming so late that the subject may have been forgotten. Say briskly what is going on.

But how, etc.

Repetitious. Good enough in a Greek tragedy where the chorus can come to the rescue in a developing footnote. Not necessary in a shorter document.

Is accomplished

Accomplish seems not only to have won World War II but to have lost the peace as well. *Do, did,* and *done* have gone from the language.

It might have been said by us

Fluffy interjection. The kind of flocculent flaking out which used to disturb Winston Churchill.

Bovine dimensions

Puddery.

High level personnel (Previously discussed)

It works well. It fails

One often sees antithetical or contradictory statements glowing side-by-side. He takes his choice. They are rarely as short and blatant as these but look out for them.

Presently

The word *presently* seems to have come to mean *now* in the same way *anymore* means *now*. One often hears "Anymore I'm going to town," about which I hardly care any more.

Feel free

There are much better ways of giving permission than to say *feel free,* but it rules the day.

Methodology

See *Usage.*

Bovine mammal

Puddery.

Is found, etc.

Passive.

Mitigation (Previously discussed)

Overall (Previously discussed)

It is not all that important

An antecedent for the stock introductory or interjected *this* or *that* has gone from the language. An obscure implication is introduced for the listener. It is rarely denotive and is so connotive that it means nothing. A common introduction to an essay today would be the words *This guy,* which neither denotes nor connotes and gets us back to the language *ugh,* the swamp talk of aborigines.

The stimulus impinging. Olfactory organs

These suggest delusions of grandeur.

Marked

Over a long period of time I have rounded up nearly a hundred synonyms for *marked* which anyone can find if he wants to come out of the jungles of clichés.

Multitude of cases

Cases sometimes implies sick people, sometimes examples, and sometimes containers for bottled whiskey. Keep your eye on *case* and *cases* and distinguish *cases* from *patients.*

Is said to seem to have gone

The bashful, weakening interjection.

Not unfresh

The cult of the obscure thrives on messing things up with double negatives.

Masculine member of the cow family

Puddery.

Sotto voce; Dolce far niente

If you use foreign or obscure words, except in scholarly papers, translate or paraphrase them for the unwary. Use them sparingly. Some scatter Latin, French, Italian, and even Greek, if they can print it, around to impress friends and confuse enemies. Use them if you feel you must, but it is pretty nice to put in the translation. It might even convert an enemy.

Be careful in cow pastures

Inclusion of scatological comments is a matter of taste. Taste is dead in much writing today. If you have good taste, use it.

Contractions, spasms, etc.

Tautology neither clarifies nor emphasizes.

Activating mechanisms to initiate

Heavy.

Neuromusculo-, etc.

The chain reaction which puts together a series of words in this fashion produces a domino effect—words leaning one on another to form one. Contract a whole paragraph into one gnarly word. Permitted in German, it does not work well in English.

So called

So called should almost always be *re*called.

That loud

See *It is not all that important.*

It hears good

This is like *a bed sleeps three.* It may be a good design for living but gives no repose to the spirit.

No noise soundwise

Perhaps users of this form of crippled English could stop their "wise"-cracks if they remembered the query of the father owl of the mother owl—"how is our little owl wisewise?"

Here is the way the ten-year-old wrote it according to Ernest Gowers.

The bird that I am going to write about is the owl. The owl cannot see at all by day and at night is as blind as a bat.

I do not know much about the owl, so I will go on to the beast which I am going to choose. It is the cow. The cow is a mammal. It has six sides—right, left, an upper and below. At the back it has a tail on which hangs a brush. With this it sends the flies away so that they do not fall into the milk. The head is for the purpose of growing horns and so that the mouth can be somewhere. The horns are to butt with, and the mouth is to moo with. Under the cow hangs the milk. It is arranged for milking. When people milk, the milk comes and there is never an end to the supply. How the cow does it I have not yet realised, but it makes more and more. The cow has a fine sense of smell; one can smell it far away. This is the reason for the fresh air in the country.

The man cow is called an ox. It is not a mammal. The cow does not eat much, but what it eats it eats twice, so that it gets enough. When it is hungry it moos, and when it says nothing it is because its inside is all full up with grass.[2]

During a period when I had a great deal of editorial responsibility, I made a special effort to see if there was anything incorrigibly innate in writing a medical paper which required it to be obscure, dry, tedious, and obtuse. The authors of such papers are generally proud of what they have done, and few will recognize the great improvement which simplifying and following the ordinary rules may bring. On the other hand, an occasional one will be delighted and a rare one will even go to the trouble of trying to learn by precept and example, by diligent practice, and by infinite repetition and rewriting to produce a clear, simple, and excellent paper. I do not know why those who express themselves vividly in conversation and indeed may delight their listeners when they fall to writing are seized with a kind of stylistic parkinsonism which makes them rigid, trembly, and given to festination in long sentences which fall down when rounding a curve or cannot stop at the proper place. The linguistic equivalent of the pill-rolling tremor characterizes much writing. They get into a strange habit pattern, acting like escapees from the kingdom of clarity. They are drugged by jargon.

I do not understand the great barrier reef which separates most doctors not from literacy but from the capacity to articulate their thoughts in writing, to arrange their ideas in orderly simplicity, and to express their thoughts in writing which goes beyond pidgin medicalese. Education in writing requires discipline; multiple and repeated efforts; and innumerable versions corrected, studied, read aloud, compressed, simplified, and maybe consigned to the flames and begun over again. In an age when multiple choice rather than essay selection has determined those who succeed and when almost no recent primary or secondary education included carefully reviewed drill in composition and grammar, it is small surprise that the journals are as bad as they are.

A codex for writing might be derived from an oversimplified synthesis of Fowler, Quiller-Couch, and Ernest Gowers with some savor of Strunck and John Livingston Lowes put in for spice. Remember that these are rules for those who have not mastered the technique. Genuises can get away with anything.

Words have a way of being abraded by too much use. Their sharp aromatic tang of freshness is removed. New words and new ways of using old words are coming in all the time. They become tics or habit patterns. They are overworked and rapidly reach a point of exhaustion or death. New words, if used with precision, accuracy, and restraint, are fine. But beware of the writer who leans on them as crutches to hold him up during spells of the empty head. Do not use clichés if you can find a good expression. Beware of *overall, structuring, decimate, substantive, ghetto, knowledgeable, simplistic, personnel, hopefully, disadvantaged, mitigate against, feel free to, dialogue, strategies, priority, and -wise*. Watch out for nouns converted into verbs and verbiage by *-ize, -ise, -age,* and the like.

Use as few words as you need to express meaning. Extra words obscure and tire the reader. Expunge superfluous adverbs and adjectives. Do not use a sentence where a single word will do. If simple familiar words express your meaning well, do not use ornate or far-fetched ones. Your reader is more likely to understand simple, old familiar words. Use words with precise denotive meaning rather than vague connotive implication. Only thus can your meaning be at once exact and clear. Concrete words have stronger and sharper meaning than abstract ones. In sum, employ simple, familiar, and precise words and omit the superfluous.

References

1. Symmers, W. St. C.: Silicone Mastitis in "Topless" Waitresses and Some Other Varieties of Foreign-body Mastitis. *British Medical Journal, 3:*19, July 1968.
2. Gowers, Sir Ernest: *The Complete Plain Words.* London, Her Majesty's Stationery Office, 1954, p. 48.